HEALING YOUR PROSTATE

Natural Cures that Work

HEALING YOUR PROSTATE

Natural Cures that Work

Eva Urbaniak, N.D.

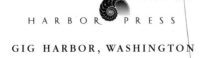

HARBOR PRESS

GIG HARBOR, WASHINGTON

Library of Congress Cataloging-in-Publication Data

Urbaniak, Eva, 1953-
    Healing your prostate: natural cures that work / Eva Urbaniak.
        p.   cm.
    Includes biographical reference and index.
    ISBN 0-936197-35-8
    1. Prostate—Diseases—Alternative treatment.   2. Naturopathy
I. Title.
RC899.U73   1998
616.6'506—dc21   98-8573
                                                             CIP

IMPORTANT NOTICE:

HEALING YOUR PROSTATE
Natural Cures that Work

Printed in the United States of America
10 9 8 7 6 5 4 3 2 1

Harbor Press, Inc.
P.O. Box 1656
Gig Harbor, WA 98335

To the memory of Dr. John Bastyr,
whose life was a living example of the truth and power
of natural healing, and whose words of inspiration
and encouragement coaxed me onto the path
of higher learning and healing.

Contents

Foreword

D R. EVA URBANIAK has written a fine book on the treatment of prostate disease. I recommend it for traditional and complementary practitioners, as well as patients and concerned family members.

True to her naturopathic-holistic background, Dr. Urbaniak addresses the effects of the environment, diet, and stress on the health of the prostate. These areas of causation are often omitted or minimized by traditional medicine. Well-outlined, easy-to-follow treatment options are provided by the author including modifying one's diet, taking specific vitamins and minerals, using reflexology techniques, and other naturopathic remedies.

This book merits attention for several other reasons as well. The first of these is that Dr. Urbaniak recognizes the importance of empowering the patient with knowledge and information, as well as removing fear from diagnosis, treatment, and the doctor-patient relationship. In addition, I compliment her highly on her chapter on mind/body medicine and the prostate. These pages show Dr. Urbaniak's wide knowledge of the healing process and her skills in taking a patient history—skills that encompass the social, psycological, and traumatic aspects of an individual's life.

As a primary care physician and psychosomatician, I have been keenly aware of the male psyche's strong propensity to focus problems of anxiety, unrecognized trauma, and fear into the area of the prostate gland. When these mind/body symptoms are not recognized as such by the practitioner, or mistakenly given a diagnosis of chronic prostatitis, costly long-term treatment with antibiotics and unwarranted diagnostic testing can easily result. This chapter closes with a number of useful mind/body techniques to reach the deeper levels of a patient's unconscious and initiate the healing process. I also commend Dr. Urbaniak's recognition of the harmful effects of negative emotions such as fear, depression, and anger on the immune system.

As a sidelight, the wisdom, skill, and caring of Dr. Urbaniak expressed towards her patients comes through in these pages. She is a true doctor of the mind, body, and spirit. Read and learn from *Healing Your Prostate: Natural Cures that Work.*

Thomas G. Pautler, M.D.
American Board of Family Practice
Fellow and Diplomat, American Board
of Medical Psychotherapists

Introduction

Y OU HAVE PICKED UP this book for a reason. Whether
you are wondering about the health of your prostate, or
your health in general, or if you are a friend or loved one of
such a person, it is very important for you to read this book.

My interest in the subject of prostate health has evolved
as a result of a high number of male patients reporting some
kind of prostate difficulty. As a naturopathic physician, I specialize in the healing of disease through natural means. Wanting to do the very best for my patients has led me to research
the subject further to find out what works and what doesn't.
In this book you will find the current successful natural
approaches for achieving and maintaining prostate health in
an easy-to-understand format. With the tools provided here,
you will be empowered to make a more informed choice
about the methods and treatments that will work best for
you, and to take charge of your own health.

The healing of disease by natural means is the central
point around which the principles of naturopathic medicine
are built. All naturopathic doctors are eclectic and are trained

in many modalities such as homeopathy, physical therapy, massage, therapeutic nutrition, and counseling. Some choose to specialize in the areas that interest them the most. But we are all united by the basic principles of naturopathy and vow to conduct our practices in adherence to our basic philosophy. To quote from the Naturopathic Physician's Oath: "According to the best of my ability and judgment, I will use methods of treatment which follow the principles of Naturopathic medicine:

First of all, to do no harm.

To act in cooperation with the
Healing Power of Nature.

To address the fundamental cause of disease.

To heal the whole person through
individualized treatment.

To teach the principles of healthy living
and preventive medicine...."

Although some of the ideas and treatments presented in this book have their roots in centuries-old medicine, modern research being conducted on natural substances and therapies has substantiated their effectiveness.

Another rapidly growing branch of medicine covered in this book is mind/body medicine, which embraces the idea that the mind has the power to heal the body. This branch of medicine has great potential in bringing humanity back into conventional medicine as it is already being successfully used in many cancer and AIDS programs, and more recently has shown great promise in treating chronic conditions such as allergies.

Greater awareness of health and health problems has brought us knowledge regarding the treatment of prostate problems. If we accept the fact that each individual has his or her own unique biochemical makeup, we also accept that what works for one may not work for others. If you have prostate symptoms, you owe it to yourself to seek a medical evaluation from a trusted urologist and a naturopath who has experience in treating prostate difficulties. After getting all the facts, you can make an informed decision about what your options are and the treatment course you would like to follow.

There are many self-care treatments that can help prostate problems in addition to what your doctor recommends. If you have been diagnosed with prostatitis, BPH (benign prostatic hyperplasia), or even prostate cancer, please read this book before undergoing any further procedures, treatments, or surgery.

Prostate Problems
and How to Recognize Them

· ANATOMY AND PHYSIOLOGY OF THE PROSTATE ·

THE PROSTATE GLAND is part of the male genito-urinary system. It is located below the neck of the bladder and it
encircles the urethra. The prostate is shaped like a chestnut
and is made up of 70 percent glandular tissue and 30 percent muscular tissue. It is enclosed in a tough fibrous sac
called a capsule, and in an adult weighs about 20 grams, and
measures about 2 × 4 × 3 centimeters.

The prostate gland plays an important role in human
reproduction. It produces and secretes a thin, milky fluid that
is an important component of semen. This fluid helps
increase the chances of fertilization because it contains nutrients such as zinc, protein, calcium, and citric acid, which
nourish the sperm, and it is alkaline, which helps to sustain
the sperm in the acid environment of the vagina.

Another important reproductive function of the prostate is

that when its muscles contract, prostatic fluid is squeezed into the urethra and out of the penis during ejaculation.

The prostate gland also secretes very biologically active molecules called *prostaglandins*, which are fatty acid derivatives that function like hormones. They stimulate the cardiovascular system and smooth muscle, and, in females, cause the uterus to contract. There are more than a dozen types of prostaglandins.

Prostate cells also produce a protein called *prostate specific antigen*, or *PSA*. PSA levels can be monitored by a simple blood test to detect the possible presence of infection or prostate cancer; a high PSA level could indicate a problem. *However, it is important to remember that PSA levels can rise from normal aging as well as from infection or cancer. A continuous, rapid, and sharp increase in PSA is what seems to suggest that a problem could be cancer rather than other conditions of the prostate.*

The prostate contributes to the discomfort felt when a man experiences prolonged arousal that does not culminate in orgasm. Fluid is secreted during arousal and if not released, exerts pressure on the prostate and testicles. A dull ache and discomfort is felt more in the testicles than the prostate because the prostate has fewer nerve endings.

• IDENTIFYING PROSTATE PROBLEMS •

The three most common problems that can affect the prostate are *prostatitis*, or inflammation of the prostate, *benign prostatic hyperplasia*, or *BPH*, and *prostate cancer*. General symptoms of a prostate problem include:

- Frequent urination, especially at night
- Difficulty with urination
- Decreased force of urine flow
- Burning with urination
- Low back and leg pain

- Sensation of a tight band around the body below the umbilicus (navel)
- Difficulty in maintaining erection during intercourse
- Sense of overall fatigue

Prostatitis

Prostatitis, or inflammation of the prostate is usually caused by an infection in the prostate gland. It can be acute (sudden) or chronic (recurring or long-standing). Symptoms of *acute prostatitis*, as the name suggests, are more severe than those of chronic prostatitis, and they include:

- Pain in the perineum, or the region between the scrotum and the rectum
- Fever
- Increased frequency of urination
- Burning with urination
- Blood or pus in the urine

Bacteria that cause acute prostatitis include E. coli., staph, and strep. Occasionally a fungus such as candida albicans, the common organism which causes yeast infections in women, can also cause acute prostatitis. Although these organisms are normal residents of the human body, any imbalance or compromise of the immune system can cause overgrowth. Sexually transmitted diseases that can cause symptoms similar to acute prostatitis are gonorrhea, trichomoniasis, and chlamydia.

Usually, it is possible to culture bacteria from prostatic fluid after it is expressed by prostatic massage. The type of bacteria that is causing the acute prostatitis can be identified by having your doctor test either prostatic fluid or urine. Acute prostatitis left untreated can be very serious. The urethra can become totally blocked, completely stopping urine flow and causing further infection, which can travel up the ureters to the kidneys.

3

Unlike acute prostatitis, which is normally caused by an easily identifiable bacterial infection, *chronic prostatitis* is very difficult to treat because its causes are usually not clear. It is a long-standing or recurring inflammation of the prostate that can be caused by bacteria or a variety of other factors that are difficult to identify. We do know, however, that it is usually not caused by a current infection. Most likely it is caused by residual inflammation and spasm from a previous infection, probably related to the urinary system, or a case of acute prostatitis.

The symptoms of chronic prostatitis are similar to those of acute prostatitis, but they are less severe and there is usually no fever. Prostatic massage has been used successfully to treat the painful symptoms of chronic prostatitis by causing the release of cellular debris and trapped fluid. This is most often done by a physician, but in some cases patients have learned to self-administer the procedure. This can be risky and awkward so I recommend that you see a physician if you need to have this done. Cultures done on the fluid from chronic prostatitis patients usually show that only inflammatory cells are present.

Sometimes chronic bacterial prostatitis can result from the presence of calculi (stones) which have formed in the prostate. The stones themselves are the source of the irritation and infection in the gland, and are usually removed along with the rest of the prostate. The cause of these stones is unknown.

Prostatodynia (Painful Prostate)

A condition that may occur simultaneously with prostatitis, or may be experienced as a separate condition, is called prostatodynia, or painful prostate. The discomfort is focused in the groin, perineum, penis, testicles, and low back. The physiological cause for the pain is muscular tension of the pelvic floor and spasms of the prostatic urethra (the portion of the urethra closest to the prostate). One of the root causes of painful prostate may be incomplete ejaculation, but there are a variety of other possible causes that should be addressed by a physician. The psychological problems associated with prostatodynia, such as anticipation of pain with arousal or with sexual relations, can have a negative impact on a man's self-esteem. Feelings about sexual performance should be discussed with a trusted professional. Self-talk related to this issue will be discussed further in Chapter 7, "Mind/Body Medicine and the Prostate: The Psychology of Healing."

Benign Prostatic Hyperplasia (BPH)

Benign prostatic hyperplasia, or BPH, is a nonmalignant (non-cancerous), abnormal enlargement of the prostate. It is very common especially after middle age; by the age of 80, 80 percent of all men have BPH. One out of eleven men with BPH will develop prostate cancer. Depending on the severity of the enlargement, symptoms vary, ranging from mild difficulty with bladder function to full-blown obstruction of the urethra which requires medical intervention. The symptoms reported by most of my patients include:

- Sensation of a full bladder even after voiding
- Nocturia, or the need to urinate several times a night
- Weakening of the urinary flow once urination has begun
- Painful urination
- Constipation, which can irritate the prostate further

If you have any of the above symptoms, and you have to urinate more often than usual, have difficulty postponing urination, or find that your urinary stream stops and starts, you probably have some degree of prostatism or BPH. Intensity and frequency of the symptoms determine severity.

The chief mechanism involved in BPH is hormonal. Here's how it works: The prostate tissue is sensitive to the hor-

mones *testosterone* and *dihydrotestosterone (DHT)*. Testosterone, which is produced by the testes, is converted to DHT
through the action of a prostatic enzyme called *5-alpha
reductase*. DHT is the hormone that causes prostate cells to
grow and proliferate.

As men age, testosterone levels begin to diminish, and
other hormones such as estrogen and prolactin increase.
Remember that men and women both produce male and
female hormones, but that testosterone is crucial to males.
Lifestyle factors that can have a profound effect on a man's
hormonal status are stress and beer drinking. Both have been
shown to increase prolactin levels. Prolactin increases testosterone activity in the prostate, thereby increasing the synthesis of DHT. More DHT in the prostate means more growth
of prostate cells.

A sobering revelation regarding prostate problems, including BPH and cancer, is that the pervasiveness of toxic chemicals, heavy metals, and pesticides in our environment may
in fact be causing these and other problems. The reason for
this may be that glandular tissue is extremely vulnerable to
these poisons.

In addition, a synthetic estrogen and harmful drug called
DES (diethylstilbestrol), which was originally banned in the
1950s from human use, is now being used in the treatment
of prostate cancer. The ban was lifted in spite of the fact that
DES caused—and is still causing—cancer in the offspring
of pregnant women who took it to prevent miscarriages.

Within the last several years, DES was implicated in a story from Puerto Rico which reported that five- and six-year-
old girls were developing breasts and menstruating. The reason for this may be that the chickens and livestock these
children are eating are routinely given DES—and have been
since the 1950s in spite of the devastating effects of this drug.
Does this not make you wonder why the ban was lifted and
who lifted it?

Prostate Cancer

Recent figures on cancer deaths have shown prostate cancer to be the number two killer of men, exceeded only by lung cancer. The National Cancer Institute admits that conventional medical treatments for prostate cancer—radiation, surgery, and drug therapy—all have major drawbacks. But the irrefutable fact is that cancer has become a part of our lives. Every person living today has either had a family member who has battled cancer, or known someone whose life has been touched in some way by cancer.

Prostate cancer is usually very slow-growing and can lie dormant for many years. Symptoms may be altogether absent or may be similar to BPH and prostatitis. The three most noninvasive tests used to evaluate the condition of the prostate are the *digital rectal exam, the PSA blood test,* and a *transrectal ultrasound scan.*

Men between the ages of 35 and 40 should have a digital rectal exam every year to screen for cancer. The exam is quick and simple, relatively noninvasive, and can give a physician a great deal of information as to the condition of the prostate.

The PSA blood test can be done starting with a baseline at age 50, and monitored periodically thereafter.

Ultrasound should be done if the digital rectal exam is positive for nodules and/or PSA is elevated.

Biopsy, although the only definitive means of confirming cancer, is invasive and risky because of the chance of spreading the cancer cells.

One patient of mine has decided to do what is called "watchful waiting." Watchful waiting is now considered a treatment option because prostate cancer rarely becomes aggressive. This can be difficult because not knowing can be stressful. In this patient's case, PSA is continuing to rise, the prostate is not enlarged, but there is a nodule present.

Regardless of which treatment options you choose, it is

important to have a good rapport with your physician. You should feel empowered making decisions regarding your health. Your doctor should be willing to discuss all tests, procedures, treatments, and their pros and cons. I would be very wary of doctors who want to operate right away, or who use tactics of intimidation. Ask questions; bring a list if you can't remember them all. Be sure to ask your doctor if he or she would support your decision regarding treatment. Does your doctor know anything at all about alternative treatments? Many doctors are now becoming enlightened to the benefits of natural therapies and can be valuable allies in your right to choose.

Now that you have a general overview of what can go wrong with your prostate, you may be asking yourself, "Am I at risk? What 'type' of man gets prostate cancer?"

Prostate cancer, BPH, and prostatitis can strike any man at any age. Sedentary as well as physically active men are equally at risk. African American men have the highest incidence of prostate cancer, and Asians have the lowest. It is interesting to note that when Japanese men move to the United States, the incidence of prostate cancer jumps to that of American men. This confirms the powerful influence of the environment and diet on your general health and, more specifically, on the health of your prostate. The next chapter focuses on dietary guidelines and other lifestyle choices for maintaining a healthy prostate.

· 2 ·

Eating for a Healthy Prostate

A s you know, your diet has a strong impact on your general health. But what you might not know is that it also has a critical and far-reaching effect on the health of your prostate. If you grab fast foods on a regular basis or eat the standard American diet (SAD)—high in fat, low in fiber, high in processed foods and those that are deep fried in rancid oils—you are increasing your risk for prostate problems in the future and possibly prolonging prostate problems you may have now.

We citizens of planet Earth have a lot going against us that for now is beyond our control. Toxic chemicals are permeating our environment and dangerous and deadly bacteria are contaminating our food and water supply; it's a wonder we even survive! But something we all do have control over is our food and lifestyle choices. We can purify or purchase our water and can cook our own food and do so properly to kill any potentially harmful bacteria. And we can certainly choose to eat and live more healthfully.

· WHAT NOT TO DO ·

A number of harmful lifestyle and dietary habits should be eliminated to prevent and/or treat any prostate disorders. Unfortunately, many are not only considered acceptable (smoking less so now), but have become staples in many men's lives. You need to know about them simply from a health standpoint, and then decide what you are willing to give up.

Here are the guidelines I believe are most important:

- *Smoking cigarettes is one habit that should absolutely be dropped.* Besides causing cancer, smoking contributes to poor circulation, which decreases the amount of life-giving blood that feeds all your organs and glands including your prostate.

- *Alcohol in all its forms should be eliminated from your diet.* Beer is especially harmful because it stimulates the production of a hormone called prolactin, which in men causes an increase of testosterone in the prostate and an increase in the production of dihydrotestosterone (DHT). This causes prostate cells to grow and contributes to BPH, or abnormal enlargement of the prostate (see Chapter 1).

- *Coffee should be eliminated from your diet.* It is a bladder irritant and is very damaging to the entire urinary system as well as many other systems of the body including the nervous, endocrine, and digestive systems.

A patient of mine, Walter J., who had BPH and had done much research on the subject, was being monitored by a urologist, and when first coming to see me, was taking many supplements, vitamins, herbs, elixirs, and anti-oxidant formulas for his condition. However, he had not eliminated his daily intake of alcohol and coffee. His condition was not improving and I was not surprised. As soon as Walter gave up his daily coffee and alcohol, he began to improve.

I know that coffee, alcohol, and tobacco are very difficult to give up for someone who has been using them for a long time, but it can be done and when the choice is health or illness, which would you choose? Because tea contains less caffeine than coffee and does not contain the alkaloids found in coffee, it can be used as an alternative, but ideally, caffeine in all its forms should be eliminated from your diet. To prevent the effects of withdrawal from caffeine, you can wean yourself off gradually. Green tea is a good substitute, and there are herbal teas on the market that mimic the flavor of black teas and are also excellent substitutes.

- *Drugs, whether prescription, over-the-counter, or recreational, have significant side effects and should be avoided.* Drug therapy should be a last resort for treating prostate conditions. (See Chapter 8.)

- *Fats in your diet should be kept to a healthy minimum.* You can use oils such as flaxseed, olive, sunflower, and canola. Fried foods should be completely eliminated from your diet. The high temperatures used in cooking these foods create cancer-causing substances.

- *Avoid using margarine.* The hydrogenated fats found in margarine contain trans-fatty acids which are unhealthy.

- *Test for food allergies.* Foods that have become allergens in your diet must also be considered. They can wreak havoc in the digestive system, the urinary system, and eventually other systems as well, playing a role in such diseases as arthritis, dermatological conditions such as acne rosacea, rashes of various kinds, and fungal infections of both an internal and external nature. A prostate patient of mine noticed an aggravation of symptoms after eating granola that contained almonds to which he was allergic. If you know you are allergic to a food, take care not to eat it. It takes self-control, but it can be done and sometimes the food can be reintroduced into the diet. There are effective treatments for allergies. Explore this with your doctor to find the best treatment for you. On average, nine out of ten patients screened have food allergies. The top ten most common allergens are cow's milk, wheat flour, soy, corn, eggs, sugar, citrus fruits, apples, pesticides, and coloring agents/additives found in processed foods.

• WHAT TO DO •

Proper nutrition is very simple: the simpler and least refined, the better. A high fiber, low fat, high complex carbohydrate, and moderate protein diet is the most wholesome and nourishing to follow. This means eating fresh (preferably organic):

- *Fruits and vegetables, which you should eat plenty of every day*

- *Whole grains like millet, brown rice, and oats*

- *Nuts in limited amounts which should be eaten*

*raw or soaked overnight, ground, and added to
your morning cereal*

- *Animal protein such as fish or naturally-grown
(without hormones or antibiotics) poultry or beef
(if you are not a vegetarian)*

- *Organic eggs and dairy products in limited
amounts if you are not allergic to them*

- *Living foods, which are sprouted seeds and
legumes that would continue living if planted.
I strongly recommend that you include living foods
in all meals, if possible. The sprouted seeds of alfalfa,
radish, buckwheat, lentils, peas, and sunflowers, not
only add color and zest to any salad or meal, they
are full of life-giving nutrients and enzymes necessary for good nutrition and digestion.*

- *Juices (freshly made), both vegetable and fruit,
which are very cleansing and energizing, and
should be drunk daily*

- *Pure water, which you should also drink lots of
every day*

- *Herb teas*

I also recommend that pumpkin seeds be included in your
diet. Pumpkin seeds are high in zinc and essential fatty acids,
nutrients necessary for a healthy prostate, and can be eaten
as snacks or included in meals.

A general rule of thumb for liquids is that they should be
drunk either 10 minutes before or 30 minutes after meals to
prevent stomach acids needed for digestion from being dilut-
ed. You may save a little of whatever you are drinking to
swallow your supplements with your meal. (See Chapter 3
on supplements.)

This is a very simple and healthful eating regime, but it requires awareness and willingness to try something a little different from the usual routine.

A word about the BEST diet to follow: Become aware of your specific nutritional needs by finding out about your own basic biochemistry. Your health care practitioner has thousands of tests that he or she can run on you, but the three that I consider most important are:

1. Complete blood analysis, which includes blood chemistry, blood count, PSA level, and blood type.

2. ELISA (Enzyme Linked Immuno Sorbent Assay) food allergy test, which identifies foods that are causing allergic reactions. This is a blood test, not a scratch test.

3. Hair analysis for mineral ratios, heavy metal toxicity, and oxidation rates. Hair analysis reveals the amount of toxic metals in your body and any accompanying abnormalities in mineral levels. These two factors are crucial to the proper functioning of all your cells. Hair analysis also shows whether you are a fast or slow oxidizer, which simply means whether you burn your food rapidly or slowly.

The blood and hair analyses give you information from which to gauge improvement over time. There also is a theory regarding eating for your particular blood type that I consider worth looking into called the D'Adamo theory. For information on eating for your blood type, see *Eat Right for Your Type* by Dr. Peter J. D'Adamo and Catherine Whitney.

The allergy test tells you which foods you are reacting to, but this does not mean that you will never be able to enjoy these foods again. There is now an allergy elimination technique that is noninvasive and really works! It is called NAET (Nambudripad's Allergy Elimination Technique; see Appendix for information). If allergies are a problem for you, look into this allergy-clearing technique. Freedom from allergies can give you a new life.

A hair analysis shows the various ratios of calcium, magnesium, sodium, and potassium in your body, which determine your oxidation rate. Your oxidation rate is the rate at which you burn your food. There are three main categories of oxidizers or burners: slow, fast, and mixed, which is the most balanced. A slow oxidizer is burning his food rather inefficiently, particularly fats and proteins, due to under-active thyroid and adrenal glands. Lean meats, poultry, fish, and eggs are excellent protein foods for the slow oxidizer, whereas beans, nuts, and seeds are not, and can slow down the slow burner even more. A slow oxidizer should derive most of his caloric intake from high quality, complex carbohydrates (all vegetables, whole grains such as brown rice, buckwheat, millet, pasta, and potatoes), and natural sugars (fruits), rather than from fats and oils, because fats and oils slow the oxidation rate.

On the other hand, a fast oxidizer needs fats and oils in his diet to help him digest more slowly. Fats and oils for a fast oxidizer provide an even source of energy. Sugar and stimulants like caffeine are particularly bad for fast oxidizers.

The sample menus that follow are designed to give you an idea of what the best diet based on your oxidation rate would look like. Here are a few simple guidelines:

- Foods may be interchanged within these menus.

- Lunch should be the largest meal, using sensible portions.

- Snacks can be eaten between meals if you get hungry.

- Dinner should be eaten before 7:00 p.m.

- Supplements are best taken with meals unless you are instructed otherwise.

- A minimum of two quarts of pure clean water should be drunk every day, more if you are active. Drink fluids between meals, or no less than fifteen minutes before or one hour after. Fluids drunk with meals will dilute stomach acid, and make digestion more difficult. You may have up to a half cup of liquid with a meal to swallow supplements.

- Remember to chew your food thoroughly. Do not gulp.

- If you drink tea, make sure it is herbal.

NOTE: If you are a vegetarian, you may need to alter your diet to include adequate protein such as eggs or fish.

• SAMPLE MENUS FOR THE SLOW OXIDIZER •

Breakfast

Two poached eggs on whole wheat toast
Juice, 4 to 6 ounces only.
(Vary the juices; grapefruit is excellent.
Try mixing cranberry with grapefruit
or inventing your own combinations.)
Tea or coffee substitute

Bowl of oatmeal (raisins or a small amount of butter
may be added) with sunflower seeds and almonds

Toasted whole wheat pita bread with natural nut butter
Juice, tea, or water

French toast with apple butter (no syrup)
Juice, tea, or water

Whole wheat or buckwheat pancakes
with apple butter (no syrup)
Juice, tea, or water

Millet cereal
Slice of lean meat, such as turkey ham
or natural sausage
Juice, tea, or water

Chicken breast
Whole grain toast
Juice, tea, or coffee substitute

Lunch

Broiled cod, 4 ounces
Tossed green salad with flaxseed oil dressing
(see recipe for dressing)
Lemonade (very little or no sugar), tea, or water

Broiled chicken breast teriyaki
Mixed steamed vegetables
Juice, tea, or water

Egg salad sandwich on whole wheat bread
Mixed salad with olive oil and vinegar or flaxseed oil dressing
Juice, tea, or water

Sliced turkey with light gravy
Peas, corn, carrots, yams, and/or salad
Juice, tea, or water

Lean meat
Vegetable soup
Juice, tea, or water

Chicken or beef enchilada or burrito
Tossed salad with yogurt dressing
Juice, tea, or water

Chili with beans and beef
Brown rice
Juice, tea, or water

Dinner

Broiled chicken
Mixed vegetables
Potatoes
Baked apple
Tea or water

Broiled red snapper
Salad
Brown rice or whole wheat bread (one slice)
Tea or water

Chicken chow mein
Cooked vegetables and Basmati or brown rice
Tea or water

Spaghetti and meatballs
Tossed salad with olive oil and vinegar
or flaxseed oil dressing
Tea or water

Leek and/or potato soup
Cabbage stuffed with meat
Salad
Fruit cup
Tea or water

Broccoli quiche
Steamed zucchini squash
Potatoes (small serving)
Tea or water

Meat loaf or veggie burger loaf
Brown rice
Vegetable soup
Tea or water

19

Snacks

A piece of fruit
Raw nuts and seeds
Whole grain crackers or a rice cake

Flaxseed oil dressing
(makes 3 to 4 servings)

Mix together these ingredients:
4 tablespoons flaxseed oil (virgin organic only)
2 tablespoons lemon juice
1 medium garlic clove (crushed or chopped fine)
pinch of salt and/or pepper

Alternate Salad Dressing

1 cup red wine vinegar
½ cup chopped fresh herbs (try basil, parsley,
tarragon, dill, thyme, or a combination)

Combine and bring to a boil, then cool and cover.
Let stand at room temperature for a couple of days.
Strain and serve over veggies or salads.
You can mix two teaspoons of plain yogurt
to this dressing for variety.

• SAMPLE MENUS FOR THE FAST OXIDIZER •

Breakfast

Two eggs with bacon
One slice of whole grain bread with butter
Milk, tea, or water

Ham and eggs
Hash brown potatoes
Milk, tea, or water

Natural sausage
One slice whole grain bread with butter
Milk, tea, or water

Oatmeal with small amount of butter
Slice of turkey ham or other breakfast meat
Milk, tea, or water

Vegetable and cheese omelet
Bacon or natural sausage
Milk, tea, or water

Smoked fish
One slice whole wheat toast with butter
Milk, tea, or water

Lunch

Beef tacos with lettuce
Tossed salad with flaxseed oil dressing
Tea or water

Hamburger patty
Green salad with flaxseed oil dressing
or olive oil and vinegar
Unsweetened lemonade, tea, or water

Chef's salad with sliced turkey, ham, and cheese,
and flaxseed oil dressing
Small whole wheat roll with butter
Tea or water

Grilled seafood
Chicken soup
Salad
Tea or water

Steamed rice, ¼ cup
Cottage cheese
Salad
Tea or water

Sardines on a bed of lettuce
One slice of whole wheat bread with butter
Tea or water

Avocado stuffed with crab meat
Tossed salad
Cheese cake (small serving)
Tea or milk

Dinner

Steak
Chicken soup
Caesar salad
Tea or water

Seafood dish
Beef broth
Baked potato (small)
Tossed salad with olive
or flaxseed oil dressing
Tea or water

Veal scallopini
Egg drop soup
Zucchini and carrots
Milk, tea, or water

Broiled lobster
Shrimp cocktail
Mixed salad
Tea or water

Pot roast
Cream of broccoli soup
Green salad
Tea or water

Tangy meat balls
Steamed cauliflower
Ice cream (small serving)
Milk, tea, or water

Snacks

Olives, Nuts, Seeds, Cold cuts
Cheese with or without crackers

I have given you some ideas for easy-to-prepare meals for the slow and fast oxidizer. I'd like to just add a word about vegetarianism. Of course, each person makes choices according to his or her own beliefs, and I respect that right, but I see many patients who are vegetarian and are having health problems as a direct result of their diet. A typical vegetarian diet is very high in copper, and as I mentioned earlier, copper can suppress immune function when it is abnormally high. Interestingly, one of the symptoms of copper toxicity is an aversion to meat. If you have doubts about your own copper levels, I strongly suggest you get a hair analysis. It is a relatively inexpensive test and can give you much information about your health status (see Chapter 2).

• SAMPLE MENUS FOR PROSTATE HEALTH •

Breakfast

Juice or fruit

Bowl of multi-grain hot cereal or oatmeal
with raisins and sunflower seeds, pumpkin seeds,
or almonds with rice or soy milk

Tea or coffee substitute

French toast with apple butter

Juice, tea, or water

Two poached eggs on whole grain toast

Juice, tea, or coffee substitute

Whole wheat or buckwheat pancakes
with apple butter

Juice, tea, or water

Lunch

*(Vegetarians: Substitute animal protein with
your choice of vegetable protein.)*

Lentil soup
Salad
Whole grain roll
Juice, tea, or water

Broiled fish
Salad with flaxseed oil dressing
Lemon water

Broiled chicken breast
Mixed steamed vegetables
Juice, tea, or water

Large mixed fruit salad
Tea or water

Dinner

....

Baked potato
Large serving of mixed vegetables
Green salad
Tea or water

....

Sliced turkey breast
Mixed vegetables
Small serving of potato
Baked apple
Tea or water

....

Vegetable soup
Meat or legume loaf
Brown rice
Salad
Tea or water

....

Chicken stir-fry
Brown or Basmati rice
Sorbet
Tea or water

Snacks

Fruit
Raw nuts and seeds
Whole grain crackers
Rice cakes

I have provided this glimpse of a sample diet to show you that eating well and healthfully is fairly easy. There are infinite combinations you can create with your foods. Make food your first medicine and you will start feeling better immediately.

· 3 ·

Supplements for Prostate Health

IT WOULD BE WONDERFUL if we could get all we need for optimal health from our food, but unfortunately, depletion of essential minerals in our soil, processing of foods, and the stress of living in the twentieth century have left many of us nutritionally challenged. Therefore, supplementation of the diet with concentrated nutrients is often necessary to bring the body back into balance, and more specifically, to treat prostate conditions.

Many strides have been made in the field of natural medicine to streamline treatment of prostate disorders. For example, there are many prostate supplement formulas on the market that include a combination of the supplements necessary to treat prostate dysfunction. (This is similar to the idea of a daily multi-vitamin formula.) If you purchase a prostate supplement formula, you need to know which nutrients should be included. Just check the label against the list of nutrients described in this chapter. Many of these formulas also contain herbs or botanical ingredients; see Chapter 4, "Healing Herbs for the Prostate," for information on how these substances promote prostate health. (You may already be on a vitamin-mineral supplement program and need only botanical support.)

A general rule about minerals: the chelated forms are absorbed much better by the body. For example, calcium carbonate and magnesium oxide, which are not chelated, are the crudest forms of calcium and magnesium, and are the least absorbable by the body. When purchasing a mineral supplement, look for the words *amino acid chelate* after the name of the mineral to indicate that this is the chelated form of that particular mineral. What a chelate means simply is that amino acids and other protein molecules are bound to a nutrient providing it with more binding sites for better absorption.

I would like to mention again that a hair analysis can provide you with a picture of mineral imbalances that may have occurred as a result of stress, dietary indiscretions, or exposure to toxins, all of which can affect prostate health. It is an extremely powerful method of understanding your own chemical imbalances (see Chapter 2).

Some labs that test for nutrient levels in the hair will also make supplement recommendations to correct the imbalances found, and I suggest that you use these labs. (See the Appendix for names of reputable labs.) Do not try to treat imbalances on your own, as direct replacement of low nutrients does not always work, nor does the elimination of a nutrient that shows up as high. For example, high zinc levels in a hair analysis often indicates excessive loss of zinc from bodily tissues indicating a need for zinc replacement, whereas low copper levels may indicate excessive copper stored in the tissues that is not being eliminated.

• MINERALS FOR PROSTATE HEALTH •

The following list describes the mineral supplements necessary for prostate health:

- **Zinc** is an essential mineral involved in prostate
  function. It is found in large amounts in a healthy
  prostate. Zinc deficiency is directly linked to prostate
  enlargement. Zinc shrinks prostate tissue that is
  enlarged by balancing hormones and inhibiting the
  enzyme 5-alpha reductase, which is involved in the
  conversion of testosterone to dihydrotestosterone
  (DHT). DHT is the hormone that causes prostate
  cells to grow and proliferate (see Chapter 1).

    If you supplement with zinc alone, and not in a
  multi-mineral formula, *never take it on an empty
  stomach* because it can cause upset.

    *Supplementary ranges recommended for prostate
  problems are from 60 to 120 mg. per day.*

- **Copper** is another essential mineral for prostate
  health, which although only necessary in trace
  amounts, aids in the absorption of zinc. In some
  cases, zinc taken alone can actually cause copper
  deficiency.

    *The recommended range for copper supplementation
  is 2 to 4 mg. per day.*

- **Selenium** is a powerful antioxidant trace mineral
  that specifically affects the reproductive system. It
  is also very effective in getting rid of toxic heavy
  metals from the body.

    *Recommended daily dosage is from 50 to 300 mcg.
  depending on individual needs. There is toxicity associated with high doses of selenium (500 mg.), but all*

selenium supplements are sold in microgram not mil-ligram dosages, so it is unlikely that you will have this problem. (In many cases, with supplementation more is not better).

- **Magnesium** is a mineral that can be helpful for prostate problems, especially if there is spasm of muscles during urination. Magnesium has a specific relaxing effect on smooth muscle in the entire body, so supplementation can have other positive side effects such as lowering blood pressure and reducing nervousness. Magnesium also aids in the absorption of vitamin B-6 (see section on vitamins), so be sure to take the recommended dosage or pur-chase a good quality multi-mineral formula with at least the minimum amount in a daily dose.

The recommended range for magnesium supplemen-tation is 400 to 1,000 mg. per day.

- **Calcium** is a macro mineral needed for healthy blood, bones, and teeth. It also facilitates nerve transmission, muscle contraction, and good per-meability of cell membranes, which all play an important role in prostate health.

The recommended supplementary range for calcium is 1,000 to 2,000 mg. per day.

• VITAMINS FOR PROSTATE HEALTH •

The following vitamins are essential for a healthy prostate:

- **Vitamin B-6** (Pyridoxine) aids in the absorption of zinc and magnesium, so it is critical for a healthy prostate. In order to maximize the absorption of B-6 and to prevent an imbalance of the other B-complex vitamins, *take a B-complex supplement daily of at least 50 mg., and 100 mg. if you under severe stress.*

- **Vitamin A** is a fat soluble antioxidant vitamin that is necessary for the normal functioning of the eyes, skin, immune system, and the bones, but it also protects the tissue linings of all organs including the lungs and the bladder. Fish liver oil has for many years been the accepted source of vitamin A, but since fish is not regulated and may be contaminated, other forms like beta-carotene, which is converted to vitamin A in the body, or vegetable sources like lemon grass, have proven to be just as effective in providing the body with vitamin A activity. (A handy mnemonic device to remember your baseline anti-aging antioxidants is ACES, which stands for vitamins A, C, E, and selenium.)

  Recommended daily dosage for vitamin A is from 25,000 to 50,000 IUs. Since there is toxicity associated with taking the fish oil form of vitamin A, the above dosage should not be exceeded if taking fish oil. The other forms are safe and non-toxic, and the dosage may be adjusted to provide adequate amounts.

- **Vitamin C** is critical as an antioxidant or immune system enhancer regardless of your specific type of prostate condition.

Take 3,000 to 5,000 mg. of vitamin C per day. Vitamin C usually needs to be taken separately, rather than as part of a prostate formula supplement.

- **Vitamin E** is essential for healthy heart function, skin protection, and reproductive health, fertility, and potency.

  Recommended dosage is from 400 to 1,200 IUs daily.

• OTHER HEALING NUTRIENTS •

Here are other important nutrients that can help heal your prostate:

- **The amino acids glycine, alanine, and glutamine** have been the focus of a number of interesting studies on the treatment of BPH. When given alone to research subjects these three amino acids produced a decrease in all BPH symptoms with no side effects.

  Recommended dosage is 400 mg. for glycine, 50 mg. for alanine, and 1,000 mg. for glutamine per day.

- **Essential Fatty Acids** are important to normal prostate function. The best EFAs are found in flaxseed oil, sunflower oil, and evening primrose oil. These good oils not only have an essential role in maintaining the membranes of every cell in your body and represent the optimal balance of Omega-3, 6, and 9 oils, but are involved in helping your body produce the anti-inflammatory, anti-cancer prostaglandins described in Chapter 1.

  Flaxseed oil can be used in the diet as salad dressing (see Chapter 2) or taken in capsule form *always as a separate supplement.* It cannot be heated or used in cooking and it should be kept refrigerated.

Recommended dosage for flaxseed oil is 3,000 to 6,000 mg. per day.

Evening primrose oil can be purchased in capsule form as well.

Recommended dosage for evening primrose oil is 500 to 1,500 mg. per day.

To review nutritional recommendations:

Supplement	Daily Dosage
Vitamin A	25,000-50,000 IU.
Vitamin B-Complex	50-100 mg.
Vitamin B-6	50-100 mg.
Vitamin C	3,000-5,000 mg..
Vitamin E	400-1,200 IU.
Zinc	60-120 mg.
Copper	2-4 mg.
Selenium	50-300 mcg.
Magnesium	400-1,000 mg.
Calcium	1,000-2,000 mg.
Glutamine	1,000 mg.
Alanine	50 mg.
Glycine	400 mg.
Flaxseed oil	3,000-6,000 mg.
Evening primrose oil	500-1,500 mg.

The supplements described in this chapter are effective for treating BPH, prostatitis, and can be adjuncts for cancer treatment. Many are combined for ease of use. For additional information or advice, check with your local health food store or naturopathic pharmacy (see Appendix).

Supplementation with nutrients that specifically impact prostate health will greatly improve your general health as well. You'll have more energy, an increased feeling of well being, and you'll live better and longer.

4

Healing Herbs for the Prostate

THE USE OF BOTANICAL MEDICINE, or plants for healing, is probably as old as humanity itself. From the beginning of time, man's intuition has led him to look at his surroundings and to use what the earth has produced, often by trial and error, crushing weeds and smelling them, digging roots, picking berries, harvesting flowers and leaves, to utilize the healing power of nature. The United States Pharmacopoeia, adopted as a standard for pharmacy in 1906, contains many plant-derived medicines. A good example is Digoxin, a cardiac stimulant, which is derived from the Digitalis lanata plant, or the common foxglove.

What I believe has happened, particularly in this last century with the advent of modern science, synthetic drugs, and the technological revolution, is that medicine has lost precious contact with its roots, which lie in nature. With health care consumers looking much more seriously at alternative medicine, it will be interesting to see what unfolds in the next century!

One of the wonders of botanical medicine is that each herb- or plant-derived substance has one or more effects on an organ or system. The following list of herbs and plant substances will give you a good idea of which herbs best serve your needs. For each herb, I provide a brief description, explanation of uses and actions, and expected results. Many of these herbs are combined together in formulas, which not only enables you to experience various benefits from one substance, but in fact, combining some herbs augments the efficacy of the individual ingredients. (See Appendix for sources of combination formulas.) Some herbs you will no doubt have heard of, and others are more obscure in the treatment of prostate problems, but nonetheless important for addressing specific symptoms.

• PROSTATE HERBS AND NATURAL SUBSTANCES •

Use the following herbs and natural substances to help heal your prostate:

- **Saw palmetto** (Serenoa repens) The berries of this palm tree are used as a tonifying agent (invigorates and strengthens) for the male reproductive system. Saw palmetto is a mild diuretic (stimulates urine excretion), a urinary antiseptic (inhibits bacterial growth), and a hormonal balancer. Now that repeated clinical studies have shown saw palmetto's efficacy in treating BPH and some infections of the genito-urinary tract, holistically-minded M.D.s and urology specialists are recommending that patients try this herb before resorting to more invasive procedures. This herbal medicine will usually shrink the enlarged prostate tissue of BPH and thus relieve many of the annoying urinary symptoms. It is best to use this herb in concentrated extract capsule form.

Avoid tinctures because they contain a much weaker form of the herb and alcohol, which I do not recommend. *Therapeutic dosage range is from 350 to 750 mg. per day, depending on the potency of the extract.*

- **Pygeum africanum** (no known common name) This plant extract comes from the bark of an African evergreen tree. In repeated clinical studies on the effectiveness of pygeum extract, there was reduction of all associated symptoms of BPH such as number of urinations at night, relief of restricted urine flow, frequency, urgency, and pain with urination. Sexual functioning was also shown to improve. In one study using 100 mg. daily, the only side-effect reported in 5 out of 263 patients was mild gastric upset. *Recommended dosage range of pygeum extract is 25 to 100 mg. per day.*

- **Bearberry** (Arctostaphylos uva ursi) This is a low-growing evergreen shrub used extensively as decorative ground cover in the Pacific Northwest. The leaves are used medicinally. Bearberry is a urinary antiseptic and tonifier, soothes the urinary system, and is quite astringent (tightens tissues and stops bleeding). Through its general supporting action on the kidneys and bladder membranes, bearberry can help with all urinary symptoms, including "dribbling".

- **Cranberry** (Vaccinium macrocarpon) Cranberries are astringent, slightly diuretic, and healing to the urinary tract. They are available in many forms such as frozen, canned, dried, juiced, and concentrated in soft gel capsules, so just include cranberries in your diet. Cranberry juice can be helpful with irritation after procedures such as cystoscopy (viewing the bladder through the urethra). Look for the unsweetened type.

• **Parsley** (Petroselinum crispum) Parsley is used extensively as a culinary herb, but it has potent medicinal effects. The entire plant can be used— leaves, stems, and root. Chiefly, it is a diuretic, helping the body get rid of excess urine, or in the case of prostate problems, residual urine. It can also be helpful in increasing the force of the urine. Parsley is also a supposed aphrodisiac, which could be helpful for impotence. Use parsley in your fresh juices, in salads, and in cooking. Parsley may be found in some combination formulas as well.

• **Siberian ginseng** (Eleutherococcus senticosus) While there are many different types of ginseng (see below for several examples), I prefer Siberian ginseng because its effects seem to be stronger and more rapid. Within just a few days, patients experience increased energy, stamina, and resistance to stress and illness.

Siberian ginseng grows only in northeast Asia, Siberia, China, and Japan, and as with all ginsengs, the root of the plant is used to make ginseng supplements in a variety of forms.

Ginseng of any type produces these similar results:

1. Helps the body and mind adapt to stress of all kinds.

2. Expands and relaxes blood vessels, which increases blood flow and volume, bringing more life-giving nutrients to your organs and glands.

3. Increases overall energy and stamina.

4. Increases resistance to illness.

5. Acts as an anti-depressant, creating a feeling of well-being.

6. Treats conditions associated with aging particularly well.

7. Acts as an aphrodisiac for some people.

In addition to Siberian ginseng, other types of common ginseng include:

• **Panax ginseng**—Also called Korean ginseng, red or white ginseng, or red Korean ginseng. Grows in China and Korea. Especially effective for helping with the recovery from any illness and improving endurance.

• **American ginseng**—Also called Panax quinquifolium. Grows in the United States. Effective for helping with the recovery from any illness and improving endurance.

• **Panax pseudo-ginseng**—Also called San qi (Tienchi) ginseng. Grown in China. Researched in China and the United States as treatment for cardiovascular conditions, high blood pressure, and high cholesterol. Particularly good for healing wounds, angina symptoms, helping with the recovery from any illness, and improving endurance.

Ginseng can be taken in many forms: tea, powder, liquid vials, capsules or blended in a formula. *Amounts considered safe are anywhere from 100 to 1,000 mg. daily. Although there is very little toxicity associated with ginseng, excessive use may raise blood pressure or cause headaches. Discontinue use if either of these symptoms occur. It is prudent to supplement in the lower range.*

- **Horsetail** (Equisetum arvense) This common herb resembles its name with its bushy hair-like stems and leaves. The aerial part is used as medicine. Horsetail is a powerful diuretic and astringent for the genito-urinary system. It is excellent for the treatment of incontinence and dribbling, reduces hemorrhage, and promotes healing because of its high silica content. It is used specifically for inflammation and benign enlargement of the prostate gland. It can be purchased in tea or capsule form. There is no toxicity associated with horsetail.

- **Hydrangea root** (Hydrangea arborescens) This is another lesser known herb but like horsetail, it is specifically used for the urinary system. It is a diuretic and it prevents kidney stones. The root is used for inflamed or enlarged prostate glands, bladder infections, and kidney stones or gravel. It can be taken as tea, or in capsule form.

- **Juniper berries** (Juniperus communis) These are the berries of the juniper tree and are used to give gin its distinctive flavor. They contain essential oils, bioflavonoids, resin, tannin, and organic acids. Juniper berries are diuretic and antiseptic, which make them excellent for treating bladder problems associated with prostate conditions. However, the essential oil present in the berries is stimulating to the kidneys, therefore juniper should be avoided when there is any kidney dysfunction.

- **Flower and bee pollen** These substances have been used for thirty years in Europe for the treatment of BPH and prostatitis with quite impressive results. Both flower pollen and bee pollen contain concentrated forms of almost all known nutrients, vitamins, minerals, anti-inflammatory substances, and free-radical scavengers (anti-aging substances that help prevent cellular damage). Pollen relaxes the muscles of the bladder sphincter, which helps with urinary symptoms. Pollen is also a very high-energy food and could correct a state of general weakness. Bee pollen is more effective for prostatitis than for BPH, but it is worth trying for both conditions. One pure flower pollen product, which was used in the European studies, is called *Cernilton*. The recommended dosage of Cernilton is four to six capsules a day, and with bee pollen, half a teaspoon three or four times a day. Both products can be taken at the same time.

• ADDITIONAL NATURAL THERAPIES •
Glandular Therapy

Glandular therapy consists of supplementation with a tablet that contains organ tissue either from bovine or porcine sources that is purified and desiccated. In the case of prostate problems, tissue of the prostate, testicles, thyroid, liver, and other organs may be used. Many naturopaths and holistic M.D.s prescribe glandulars to support specific organs and systems being treated. Strict vegetarians would object to using such a product, but the fact that glandulars work cannot be refuted. Glandular support formulas are available at your local health food store or natural pharmacy. Take as directed.

Homeopathy

Fnally, because homeopathic medicine is so popular internationally, and because homeopathic remedies are made from natural vegetable, mineral, or animal sources, I thought it was important to mention it in this chapter.

Homeopathy is the administering of highly-diluted substances which, if taken in larger amounts, would mimic the presenting symptoms. These substances stimulate the body's own defense system and bring it back into balance.

Homeopathic remedies are usually prescribed by a practitioner because objectivity is extremely difficult when prescribing for oneself. Because choosing a remedy simply on the basis of one symptom does not follow homeopathic principles, usually several symptoms are taken into consideration before a remedy is prescribed.

The homeopathic version of the herb Digitalis, mentioned at the beginning of this chapter, is one of the remedies prescribed for prostate problems, but Digitalis is only available through practitioners of homeopathy. So if homeopathy is something you would like to explore, I encourage you to seek out a practitioner in your area.

· 5 ·

Home Hydrotherapy
for Healing the Prostate

HYDROTHERAPY, OR THE USE of water in all three of its forms
—liquid; solid, as ice; and gas, as steam—has been used
for healing since the seventeenth century. It actually goes
much further back to ancient Greece when the followers of
the goddess Hygeia established guidelines for healthful living.
This is the origin of the word hygiene. Water was also used
for healing in ancient China, Egypt, Rome, Persia, and India.

Modern hydrotherapy has evolved from many influences,
from orthodox medical doctors to unschooled peasants,
priests, and so-called "hydropathists," or hydrotherapists,
which is what proponents of hydrotherapy were called up
until the late 1800s.

At the turn of this century, sanitariums and hospitals still
used hydrotherapy as an established treatment, and in European countries today, water treatments are used pre-opera-
tively to boost the immune systems of patients. Naturopathy
is one discipline that has retained the use of hydrotherapy

in healing, embracing the philosophy of treating the whole person using non-invasive techniques.

Many different kinds of hydrotherapy techniques are used for the purpose of healing. A few treatments can actually be done in the privacy of your own home and can help for conditions of the prostate. It is important to remember that poor circulation contributes to many conditions of ill health, including prostate dysfunction. Because water is an excellent conductor of heat and cold, it can have profound positive effects on circulation and health.

Water treatments today consist of steam baths, hot and cold compresses, sitz baths, alternate baths, ice packs, poultices, enemas, colon irrigations, wet sheet packs, cold mitten friction rubs, and hydrotherapy combined with electrotherapy, botanical medicine, and nutrition.

Of course, steam baths, hot tubs, and saunas are readily available in places such as health clubs, gyms, or apartment complexes, and can be helpful for relaxation, maintaining healthy skin, and detoxification. Even if you prefer to shower, you might try taking more hot baths because immersing the lower half of your body in warm to hot water has a profound effect on blood flow to the prostate and surrounding structures. Also, finishing a bath with a cool shower is not only stimulating to the circulatory system, but to the endocrine system as well. In fact, just about every hydrotherapeutic procedure ends with a cold or cool rinse of the area treated. This works as a vascular pump causing the blood vessels to contract and move the blood.

• THE ALTERNATE HALF-BATH OR SITZ BATH •

The alternating sitz bath is very effective for prostate problems. Since no one has specially designed sitz baths in the home, we will adapt the procedure to allow you to do it yourself. This is called the alternate half-bath or sitz bath.

You will need:

- Bathtub filled approximately one-third with hot water (106-110° F)

- Bath towel and hand towel soaking in a basin containing cold water (55-75° F)

- Bath thermometer (optional)

- Dry towel or blanket to cover back and shoulders, if necessary, to keep you warm. If possible, bathe in a warm area. It is important not to get chilled during the treatment.

- Dry towel on edge of bathtub to sit on

- Watch or timer

1. Fill your bathtub with hot water, just enough to cover your body up to your navel. Have everything ready before you get in. The basin with the cold water and towels should be within your reach as you sit in the tub.

2. Sit in the tub for at least three to five minutes. Then stand up, remove the larger cold, wet towel from the basin and apply it to your abdomen and genital area like a diaper.

3. Sit on the edge of the tub, keeping your feet in the water. Take the smaller cold, wet towel and apply it to your inner thighs, halfway between your knee

and groin (the reflex area for the prostate; see illustration on page ___). Do this for thirty seconds to one minute only. If necessary to prevent chilling, cover your shoulders with a dry towel.

4. Sit back in the tub again putting the towels back into the cold water.

5. Repeat this procedure two more times, *ending with a cold shower or by pouring the cold water from the basin over the areas bathed in hot water.*

6. Lie down and rest for one half-hour after this procedure, or do it before retiring.

You can modify the sitz or half-bath with your shower nozzle, especially if you have a hand held model:

1. Repeat Step 1, and then sit in the tub for at least five minutes.

2. Stand up in your bathtub and spray cold water over the lower part of your body for one minute.

3. Then sit back in the tub and make sure you bring the temperature back up to the recommended range. Let some of the water out of the tub to keep it at the same level.

4. Repeat the cold shower two more times, always alternating with the hot soak for five minutes, and always ending with a cold water rinse.

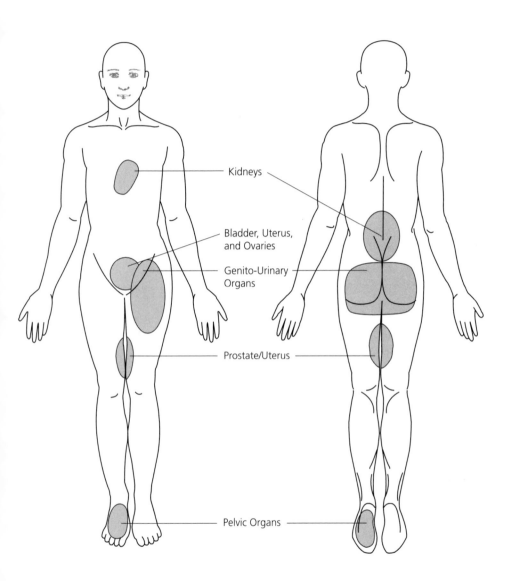

Kidneys

Bladder, Uterus, and Ovaries

Genito-Urinary Organs

Prostate/Uterus

Pelvic Organs

REFLEX POINTS FOR HYDROTHERAPY

• THE MODIFIED PERCUSSION DOUCHE •
(OR "BLITZ GUSS" / "LIGHTNING BATH")

If you have a shower massage with a hand held unit you can do a modified percussion douche. (Note: The word douche has a special meaning here; it simply means a stream of water directed against a part of the body.)

1. Set your shower massage so you are getting the strongest steady stream possible. Starting with your right foot, move the shower stream up and down your entire leg. Then go to your left leg, moving up and down and over both buttocks. Continue moving the stream of water up your back to your shoulders, arms, and neck. (This requires some agility if you're doing it yourself). *Always direct the water flow from the limbs towards your heart.*

2. Start with warm water and end with cold or cool water, whichever you can tolerate. Although this is very invigorating, it is also very stimulating to the lymphatic circulation, so lie down and rest after the procedure. (Your lymphatic system is situated alongside your venous system and is involved in combating infection and purifying the blood. Stimulating the lymph can help your body rid itself of unnecessary congested cellular debris and improve your overall health and the health of your prostate.)

This modified form of the "Blitz Guss" or "Lightning Bath" is effective for congestion of all kinds, constipation, drug addiction, and alcoholism.

• GUIDELINES FOR AT-HOME SITZ BATHS AND DOUCHES •

Hot	**Cold**	**Alternate**	**Neutral**
106-110° F	*55-75° F*	*Hot and Cold*	*92-97° F*
pain	constipation	pelvic congestion	acute cystitis
spasm	bedwetting	hemorrhoids	excitement: sexual mental
hemorrhoids	BPH	fissures	
neuralgia: testicular lumbar sciatic	incontinence due to BPH	prostatitis	
	insomnia	constipation	

Duration:

5-8 min.	5-8 min.	15-20 min. total 3-5 min. hot 30-60 sec. cold	15 min-2 hours

For prostatitis, an essence made of chamomile tea added to the hot water when doing the alternate sitz bath is stimulating to the prostate.

> ### • CONTRAINDICATIONS FOR SITZ BATHS AND DOUCHES •
> ### (OR WHEN **NOT** TO DO)
>
> | Hot | Cold | Neutral |
> | --- | --- | --- |
> | hemorrhage | heart problems | weak heart |
> | pelvic congestion | severe debility | eczema |
> | heart disease | pain | |
> | hypertension | spasm | |

In general, the direct therapeutic effects of water applications according to temperature and time are as follows:

- Hot is relaxing

- Cold is tonifying

- Neutral is calming

There aren't any health conditions that can be worsened by the neutral bath other than those presented in the above chart. Note that for acute cystitis or bladder infection (first chart), the neutral bath is used because strong changes in temperature, either hot or cold, can make an already painful condition temporarily worse. For chronic bladder problems, the alternate bath may be used. The neutral bath is very sedating so it should not be done by those with cardiac weakness. Also, it can irritate skin problems that are made worse by water, like eczema, psoriasis, and other rashes.

• THE HOT FOOT BATH •

Another very effective yet extremely simple treatment you can do at home is the hot foot bath. The mechanism involved in the hot foot bath is one called the *derivative effect*. Relief is brought to a congested organ or area (as in congestive prostatitis, or generalized pelvic congestion) by diverting blood to a distant part of the body.

The hot foot bath requires a basin with hot water (106-110° F). Simply immerse your feet for 10 to 30 minutes just above your ankles.

A variation of this treatment is to apply a hot water bottle or even a heating pad to your feet while lying in bed.

A cool compress applied to the pelvic area during this treatment increases the derivative effect. *Do not use the hot foot bath if you have any condition in which there may be loss of sensation to the extremities like diabetes, or peripheral vascular disease such as Buerger's disease, arteriosclerosis, or deep vein thrombosis.*

• THE HALF-BODY PACK •

A lower half-body pack is another treatment in which you place a thick hot moist towel across your lower abdomen and pubic area for 15 minutes. Then, you vigorously rub the heated, reddened area with a cold sponge for 2 to 3 minutes.

Repeat the whole process 3 times, always ending with the cold sponge rub.

The purpose of the half-body pack is specifically to stimulate the circulation to the pelvis.

• GENERAL EFFECTS OF WATER •

In summary, the effects of general applications of water are as follows:

Cold Water of Short Duration
1. Raises body temperature
2. Increases activity in the skin
3. Raises blood pressure
4. Contracts the muscles
5. Strengthens the heart action
6. Stimulates the nervous system
7. Stimulates metabolism
8. Slows and deepens breathing

Hot Water of Prolonged Duration
1. Raises body temperature
2. Increases activity in the skin
3. Lowers blood pressure
4. Relaxes the muscles
5. Quickens and weakens the heart action
6. Stimulates metabolism
7. Quickens and weakens breathing

Very Hot Water of Very Short Duration
1. Lowers body temperature
2. Decreases activity of the skin
3. Has no noticeable effect on blood pressure
4. Stimulates the nervous system
5. Contracts the muscles
6. Quickens and strengthens heart action
7. Contracts the surface blood vessels
8. Stimulates breathing

Local applications produce local effects similar to those of general applications. For instance, a prolonged hot application over the heart would increase and weaken the heartbeat, while a prolonged cold application would diminish and strengthen the heartbeat. A very hot short local application over muscles would relax them and dilate the blood vessels; a very prolonged cold local application would contract the muscles and constrict the blood vessels. A prolonged hot local application on the spine would lower the blood pressure, while a prolonged cold local application over the spine would raise it.

Very short, very cold local applications produce effects similar to cold applications, but more pronounced. Local prolonged hot applications and very prolonged cold applications are useful for relieving pain.

There are a great many kinds of baths, the names of which indicate their character, manner of application, or the part of the body to which they are applied.

• ENEMAS AND COLONIC HYDROTHERAPY •

Hot retention enemas have proven helpful for prostatitis. Only a small amount of water is infused at a time, held for as long as comfortably possible, and repeated several times during one treatment. If you choose to try this at home be sure that the water is not too hot. A reasonable temperature is 95° to 100° F.

Colonic hydrotherapy can be helpful for BPH, especially if hemorrhoids are a problem. If the prostate enlarges too much, constipation can become a problem and can make it difficult to have a normal bowel movement. If you have never had colonic hydrotherapy or taken any fiber supplementation, you may need a series of three or four colonic sessions to note any significant changes and/or relief. If you have a problem with constipation and/or hemorrhoids, and enemas or colonics are just not something you want to try, purchase a good fiber supplement that contains psyllium seed at your health store or naturopathic pharmacy. Psyllium seed is an excellent stool softener and detoxifying substance for the colon.

• SKIN BRUSHING •

Another excellent detoxifying technique that is extremely stimulating to the lymphatic circulation is skin brushing. Your skin is the biggest organ of your body and is involved in respiration and the elimination of wastes. Skin brushing can be done before any hydrotherapy procedure or by itself, although it seems logical to do it just prior to showering because the brushing loosens so many dead skin particles and you would want to wash them away.

Simply purchase a natural bristle fiber brush and brush your skin vigorously before doing any hydrotherapy procedure. *Always brush from your extremities towards your heart, one way only, with long, even strokes.* I had one patient who stopped drinking his morning coffee because this procedure woke him up far better.

I hope that this chapter has provided you with some hands-on techniques for treating your prostate problems at home with hydrotherapy, a type of treatment that has been used with great success for centuries. I encourage you to try these techniques and note how much better you feel.

6

Reflexology Techniques for the Prostate

REFLEXOLOGY, OR ZONE THERAPY as it is also called, operates on the premise that all the organs, glands, and nerves in your body have specific corresponding reflex areas, or points, on your toes, ankles, and the soles of your feet, as well as on your wrists and the palms of your hands.

Pain or tenderness in any of the reflex areas is a sign of congestion or malfunction in the corresponding organ or gland. Pressure or massage applied to the painful spot sends a surge of energy or stimulation to the area needing it, clearing out congestion and restoring normal function. Reflexology techniques, although very potent and powerful tools for healing, are not a replacement or substitute for medical care by a physician when it is necessary, but this simple manipulation of points on the hands and feet can do much to help relieve the tension, stress, strain, and pain that can occur as a result of modern living, and can help heal specific health conditions such as prostate dysfunction.

Many chronic cases of disease and illness which have not

responded to conventional therapies are greatly improved or eliminated with the use of reflexology. I have witnessed cases of truly miraculous healing by simply holding points on patients' feet. Many physicians, massage therapists, and practitioners of Shiatsu use these techniques successfully when treating patients. But the great thing about reflexology is that you can administer it to yourself! There is no expense, no special equipment, and nothing special to buy.

Again, I want to emphasize that although you can find a practitioner of reflexology to work on you, this is absolutely something you can administer to yourself, or have a family member help you with. One of the benefits of having someone do it for you is that you can lie down comfortably and relax, whereas doing it yourself requires attention and some expenditure of energy, and may put you in some odd positions when reaching for the feet.

In this chapter I'll share with you the major points that can help restore your prostate back to health. Use the illustrations presented as your guide.

• THE PROSTATE POINTS •

The reflex points for the prostate gland and testes reside on the inner side of the upper heel, halfway between the ankle and the base of the heel. Directly opposite on the outer side of the heel, there is an indirect reflex zone which stimulates the pelvic lymphatic channels (remember, the lymphatic system filters and cleanses the blood), and has an effect on all organs of the reproductive system. So when grasping the heel, I recommend you apply pressure to both sides. This will augment the benefits of the massage. The effect and sensation of massage in this area is so immediate and so profound that you might want to be sitting comfortably on your bed, or in such a way that you can completely relax afterward to experience the energy surge.

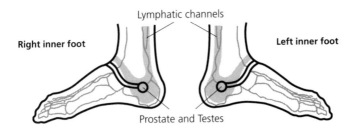

Lymphatic channels

Right inner foot

Left inner foot

Prostate and Testes

1. Place your foot across your lap, or any place where it can be easily and comfortably reached while sitting. You can sit anywhere—on your bed, in front of your computer, or wherever you are most comfortable.

2. For your right foot, grasp your heel with your left hand, for your left foot, grasp your heel with your right hand. Or if you are sitting in a chair, reach down and "pinch" your heel with the thumb and forefinger of the same hand. The thumb and forefinger are best to use to apply pressure. The pressure should be firm and steady; use a smooth milking motion upward from the base of your heel towards your ankle bone.

3. Be sure to cover the entire area of the heel below the ankle, paying more attention to the very tender places. After you have stimulated these tender spots, you will notice that they are not as sore the second time around.

4. There are other points in this region that correspond to muscles, blood vessels, organs, and glands of the pelvic cavity, so using a milking action will assure that you cover them all. You can also massage the achilles tendon with your thumb using firm pressure, then releasing completely, and applying pressure again. Do this two or three times.

Massage regularly, but lightly at first. Always massage the reflexes of both feet, as glands reside on both sides of the body. Nature's healing forces activate very quickly with this technique. I find it very interesting that Mother Nature has placed these reflexes above and away from the soles of the feet, perhaps as protection to prevent over-stimulation from walking.

A patient of mine, Dan B., who had just had prostate surgery and was in pain, was greatly relieved when I held and massaged the corresponding points to the prostate on his feet. Another patient, who had mild, chronic prostatitis, and whose prostate was congested and enlarged only on the left side, responded by saying that only the left foot reflex points were tender when massaged.

Sometimes reflex points can be sore from the scarring of any of the pelvic organs because of infection, surgery, or trauma. A current patient, Roger D., a man in his early 40s, and not a prostate patient per se, has some significant tenderness in this region which was discovered during therapeutic massage sessions. He survived a motorcycle crash six years ago, and without going into great detail here, he not only underwent exploratory pelvic surgery to rule out internal injuries, but he sustained direct blow trauma to the groin. So, although this patient is now healthy, the tenderness he is experiencing is calling attention to the area. Since he has no prostate symptoms, he is not concerned, but at some point soon, he should have a prostate check with a baseline PSA test.

Since the view of holistic medicine is to treat the whole person rather than isolated symptoms, I suggest that you massage points that relate to other organs in the body, particularly those of the urinary system, in addition to the prostate points. Therefore, I am also including here reflexology techniques for the kidneys and bladder.

• THE KIDNEY POINTS •

The kidney reflex point is on the sole of your foot, toward the center, about one inch in from the arch.

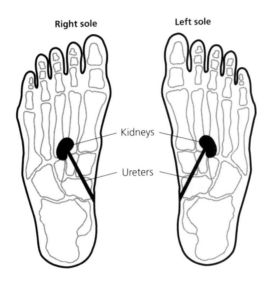

1. The best approach to massaging the kidney point is to place your foot on your lap. This time use the thumbs of both hands with a deep pressure, holding the top of your foot in place with the fingers of both hands. This part of the foot is more fleshy, so the pressure can be greater than for the ankle region.

2. Press in a circular pattern around the whole area, noting any particular points that are more sore than others.

3. Spend one or two seconds on each point, making at least two complete circular passes over the area.

4. Stretch your foot out, relax, and notice how different it feels from your other foot.

5. Repeat this same procedure on your other foot.

• THE BLADDER POINTS •

The reflex points for the urinary bladder are on the inner side of your heel below your ankle bone.

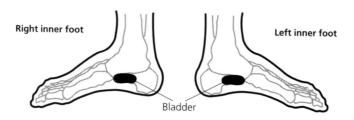

Right inner foot   Left inner foot

Bladder

1. As with the other techniques presented here, place your foot in the most accessible position for you to reach your inner heel.

2. With the thumb of whichever hand is more comfortable, place firm pressure on the inner heel, moving point-by-point upward toward the ankle bone.

3. Be aware of any tender points and go back to them spending one or two seconds on each.

4. Notice how your foot feels after the treatment.

5. Repeat this same procedure on your other foot.

Reflexology can be an excellent way to support and promote the health of your prostate. General massage for the rest of your body might also help teach you how to relax more fully, something that is essential to healthy living.

7

Mind/Body Medicine and the Prostate: The Psychology of Healing

MIND/BODY MEDICINE is the integration of body, mind, emotions, and spirit when treating a patient.

The concept of the mind/body connection has become more and more widely-accepted in medicine in recent years. Many physicians acknowledge this intangible aspect of healing. I have always preferred to call this concept mind/body unity because the word connection suggests that the two parts are disconnected. Of course, we know you cannot literally separate your mind from your body, but some patients have disconnected (disassociated) themselves from physical warning signs because of conscious or unconscious repression or suppression. A good example is high blood pressure, the silent killer. A man may be under significant stress, but ignore subtle body sensations: He gets headaches, takes aspirin, and is then surprised on a routine visit to the doctor that he has high blood pressure.

Only recently has medicine addressed the very powerful influence that a person's thoughts, emotions, and spiritual attitudes have on the physical body. I strongly believe that it is the reintegration of these parts of the "disconnected" person that is one of the most powerful aspects of true healing.

In the case of prostate difficulties, mind/body medicine plays an important role. Think of a concept introduced earlier in Chapter 5—congestion. On the physical level, prostatitis, BPH, and prostate cancer are linked to increasing amounts of congestion. Congestion leads to obstructive disease. Poor flow of blood and body fluids causes collection of toxins, which can become a knotted mass that can eventually become malignant. Similarly, negative attitudes and emotions, anxiety, depression, anger, or despair can obstruct the psyche and prevent the flow of energy needed for healing. Norman Cousins, Ph.D., author of many books including *Anatomy of an Illness* and *Head First: The Biology of Hope*, states that panic, depression, hate, fear, and frustration can have negative effects on human health, and that hope, faith, love, the will to live, purpose, laughter, and festivity can help fight serious illness.

Some of the possible mind/body issues that contribute to congestion in the area of the prostate are:

- Sexual repression (stifling sexual urges)

- Too much sex or not enough
  (and the associated feelings)

- Very tight perineal muscles (the muscles between the scrotum and the anus) due to emotional issues and the inability to relax

- Sexually transmitted diseases
  (and the associated feelings)

- Denial (conscious or unconscious) of childhood traumas which can cause dysfunction later in life

- Stress, and particularly one's relationship to stress

As I mentioned in the example of high blood pressure, stress is probably the single most important factor in determining who gets sick and who doesn't. How you react to and deal with stressful situations can determine your overall health. Just think about the last time you got sick with a cold or flu, or just felt completely run down. Then think about what was going on just prior to your illness. Your immune system responds to your brain, nervous system, and emotions. But luckily, your immune system also has the ability to learn and adapt.

A patient of mine, John D., 65 years old, has made remarkable progress in overcoming what was diagnosed by his M.D. as prostatitis. When he first came to me he was very nervous, but also very fearful of putting himself in the hands of a surgeon once again. He already had one biopsy that showed nothing six months before our visit, and was being coerced by his doctor to have another because his PSA levels had continued to rise. He was adamant about not having another biopsy, was doubtful if the prolonged antibiotic treatment he received had even helped, and wanted some alternatives. His blood pressure was elevated, he was 40 pounds over his normal weight, and had several stressful situations going on in his life. He expressed anger about living in fear since the problem first showed up two years ago. He kept a logbook of his many visits for PSA draws, digital exams, antibiotic treatments, and was feeling fed up with that, too.

John's fear and frustration about his prostate difficulty was blocking the proper functioning of his immune system. We employed many of the healing approaches described in previous chapters, but most importantly, we taught John how to *relax, let go, and go inside* of himself, and in his case, to find that warrior part of himself that did "battle" with this problem. Visualization was a powerful tool in helping John overcome his problem. Meditation, massage, and self-hypnosis were also used to help get him out of the fight or flight stress mode, and to allow his body to adapt to and recognize zero stress.

Today, only three months later, John is thirty pounds lighter, looks and feels fifteen years younger, has no symptoms, and his PSA is normal. Using the mind/body approach proved to be very effective.

Another patient, Stan B., 40 years old, came in reporting many vague symptoms. When interviewed, he disclosed that he had engaged in an extramarital affair and felt very guilty about it. All the necessary tests were run, and when I met with him again to go over the results and to see how he was doing, he reported that all symptoms had disappeared after our first visit. In his case, he just needed someone to listen and be there for him while he worked through his guilt feelings about what he had done.

Another BPH patient, Henry D., was full of anger and hatred for his wife who was addicted to drugs and was stealing from him. Although I referred this patient to another doctor closer to his area, I did check back with him and his symptoms and his problem had remained the same. Anger and hate were blocking his healing process.

If you want true healing, the mind/body approach is the most effective. Often, the blocks to healing remain until there is a shift in consciousness. Dr. Deepak Chopra, pioneer of mind/body medicine, states, "When the mind shifts, the body cannot help but follow."

• MIND/BODY TECHNIQUES •

Here are some effective techniques for helping yourself with mind/body medicine:

- **Meditation**—Explore learning some form of meditation. Research studies have shown that meditators are much healthier than non-meditators, are hospitalized less often, and have 50 percent less incidence of all categories of tumor. Meditation stills the mind and allows you to consciously observe the workings of your "computer brain" (which is constantly sifting through information) without getting caught up in the thoughts themselves.

- **Relaxation therapy**—Learn how to relax. You may also have to re-learn how to breathe deeply. So many patients I see breathe from the uppermost part of their chests, practically from their throats! Take a couple of deep breaths into your abdomen next time you're stuck in traffic and in a hurry to get somewhere, and just notice how much calmer you feel. Living in constant anxiety, fear, or tension is extremely detrimental to your health. If you need help getting started, find a hypnotherapist, counselor, or instructor who can help you devise something that will work for you. Sometimes personalized audiotape recordings are made to help bring about deep relaxation.

- **Healing affirmations**—Your subconscious mind takes in all the messages you have ever given yourself through your own internal dialogue or self-talk, and messages sent to you from others. In other words, you are programmed to think and feel a certain way. In order to change that programming, you have to feed your subconscious mind new messages, and do so repeatedly over time to manifest any change. The general rules for affirmations are as follows:

1. They must be in present tense so that the mind acknowledges that it is happening now, not at some unknown point in the future.

2. They must be positive—without any "nos," "nots," "shoulds," or "shouldn'ts."

3. They must be specific regarding the desired outcome. Ask yourself: What do I want?

Here are some examples of healing affirmations. Some are more general and others are more specific. You can certainly create an affirmation that is especially for you and your situation.

I have the power to heal now.

I radiate good health and vitality.

I have unlimited potential.

I inhale love and exhale fear.

I forgive myself now.

I have plenty of time today. (Especially good for high-stress, on-the-go types of people.)

These are affirmations for generating healing and loving feelings towards yourself and others. You can be more specific regarding any prostate problems, but it is always good to include the rest of yourself as well.

Louise Hay in her best-selling book, *You Can Heal Your Life*, offers these affirmations specifically related to the prostate:

I accept and rejoice in my masculinity.

I love and approve of myself. I accept my own power. I am forever young in spirit.

And in the case of cancer of any kind:

I lovingly forgive and release all of the past. I choose to fill my world with joy. I love and approve of myself.

Your thoughts have powerful effects on you and your world. Be good to yourself, do some life "housecleaning" to free yourself from unnecessary stress and strife. For example, choose to be around people who love and support you, rather than criticize and tear you down. And most importantly, don't let fear take hold of you in any dealings with doctors; regardless of the diagnosis, remember that *you* have ultimate control over what happens to your body. Get a second opinion if you don't feel comfortable with what your doctor has told you. Dr. Chopra's definition of quantum healing is "the ability of one mode of consciousness (the mind) to spontaneously correct the mistakes in another mode of consciousness (the body)."

Beyond body and mind is spirit. The ultimate purpose for life is spiritual growth. This consists primarily of losing our fears and learning to love unconditionally. As far as we know, only the human species knows that it will die. Awareness of our mortality forces us to consider questions of ultimate meaning, and it is usually a life-long search. So mind/body healing is actually body/mind/spirit integration, and these three aspects of the human condition are so completely intertwined, that one cannot be diseased without affecting the others.

The true meaning of holistic healing is to make whole (integrating the parts), and the word holistic comes from a root word meaning holy, suggesting that there is something sacred about healing. When I use the word sacred, I am speaking more of spirituality than religion per se, because religions are man-made, organizational expressions of the search for meaning. Spirituality, on the other hand, is a characteristic of being human. I have a great respect for this "sacred something" and attempt to access it with all patients willing to explore their potential for good health in body, mind, and spirit. This is something I sincerely wish for you.

· 8 ·

Health and Healing with the Comprehensive Approach

A COMPREHENSIVE APPROACH to healing takes into account all aspects of your physical, emotional, and psychological well-being, rather than focusing exclusively on an organ that appears to be malfunctioning—in this case the prostate—or a specific symptom. For true healing to occur, the whole person must be considered to accurately determine individual needs, and the most appropriate and effective treatment options. Your diet, lifestyle, habits, emotional makeup, and everyday attitudes all play a critical role in the health of every organ and system in your body, including the prostate gland.

I cannot emphasize enough the great impact the health of your body as a whole has on the health of your prostate. Visualize your potential high-level wellness as a germinating seed. If you plant this seed in rich, healthy soil it will grow and flourish, but if you plant it in a wasteland devoid of nutrients, it is doomed to wither and die. A body suffering from vitamin or mineral imbalances or deficiencies, parasitic infestations, improper diet, or heavy metal toxicity cannot possibly support the health of individual organs such as the prostate until these obstacles are removed and/or corrected.

• GETTING THE WHOLE PICTURE •

A comprehensive approach to healing must begin with the proper testing to get a complete picture of your health. Various blood tests and hair mineral analyses are among the tests used to determine your uniquely individual makeup and health needs. See Chapters 1 and 2 for a discussion of these tests.

Once you have the test results, a comprehensive plan must be created to get you back on the path to wellness. This plan should be based on your individual needs—rather than the commonplace "recipe book medicine" or shot-in-the-dark treatments—and should include specific dietary and nutritional guidelines, recommendations for supplementation, a lifestyle plan, counseling, if necessary, and other natural treatments that may be appropriate. All the support you need to help you reach your optimum level of health and wellness should be made available to you.

Detoxification: A Critical First Step

Let's face it. We are living in an increasingly toxic world. We have already briefly discussed the condition of our water supply, tainted meat, and other serious health challenges of our modern world. It is inevitable that each one of us, to one degree or another, will be affected by the toxins in our environment.

Whether you appear to be healthy or are being challenged by serious illness, detoxification is one of, if not the most important step in regaining or maintaining your health.

Detoxification occurs in several steps: The first step is to remove the offending substance, whether it's a plugged up, toxic colon in need of cleansing, or exposure to heavy metals, or a diet and lifestyle that perpetuates chronic illness. The next step is to rebuild and heal the afflicted tissue or system in a way that will keep it healthy over time. This includes providing it with the proper high-quality nutrition.

Unfortunately, conventional medicine, with its multi-billion-dollar focus on pharmaceuticals, has little or nothing to offer in the area of detoxification. Pharmacuetical drugs, the conventional treatment of choice, place a heavy burden on the liver, one of the main organs necessary for detoxification.

I'd like to share with you the story of a recent health disaster that involved toxic waste and the deaths of many innocent people.

Recently, an associate and I became involved in the plight of a group of farmers in eastern Washington who, because of failing health, failing crops, the death of cattle and even some family members from cancer, strongly suspected that they might have received some contaminated fertilizer. For several months after doing their hair analyses (which were all grossly abnormal, laden with toxic heavy metals), we contacted doctors who could serve as expert witnesses, attorneys, alerted the local newspapers and attempted to get the government to do something.

What culimnated from all of this was a successful lawsuit against a company that was selling toxic industrial waste as "fertilizer." Five ongoing front page articles in *The Seattle Times* exposed this outrage and brought it to public awareness. This eventually led to the passage of a state law mandating the regulation of fertilizers. It was a great victory, but it came too late for those who died early deaths as a result of the toxic load which their bodies could not eliminate.

While we were involved in this case, we discovered something very frightening and alarming: This means of toxic waste disposal has been going on for the last twenty years in at least thirteen states! Circumstances such as these very definitely contribute to the increase in cancer we are now seeing, including prostate cancer. Our bodies were simply not designed to be storage houses for toxic metals and chemicals!

In the case of heavy metal detoxification, accumulation of lead, cadmium, mercury, arsenic, aluminum, and other metals can be detected through hair mineral analysis. These can be gradually displaced and eliminated from bodily tissues by certain detoxifying nutrients administered in precisely the correct dosages.

One example of a nutrient used for detoxification is the powerful anti-oxidant *reduced L-Glutathione*, which works especially well in eliminating many toxic heavy metals such as lead, nickel, mercury, arsenic, and copper. Although copper is not considered a toxic metal and is beneficial in small amounts, in large amounts it can cause many health problems including immune system suppression, infections, and cancer. Some physicians who are aware of the importance of hair tissue analysis, have called copper the "scourge of the late twentieth century" because in the last fifty years or so copper piping was introduced, and has been used extensively ever since in homes and buildings of all kinds. Just as lead plumbing was implicated in the fall of the Roman empire, copper plumbing could be doing the same to modern society. Interestingly, a zinc deficiency can cause copper levels to rise, as can a strictly vegetarian diet.

A specifically tailored supplement program and diet, and taking very powerful substances like *reduced L-Glutathione* can speed the elimination of toxic heavy metals. *Reduced L-Glutathione should not be used in cases of insulin-dependent diabetes, severe intestinal candidiasis (yeast infection), and cystinuria (elevated levels of cystine in the urine).*

• PROSTATE CANCER •

Perhaps the most dramatic example of the importance of a comprehensive approach to healing is in the case of cancer. After seeing many patients with varying levels of prostate disease including prostate cancer, I am convinced that cancer is not something that just "happens." It is the end result or the manifestation of underlying problems that affect the body adversely, usually over a long period of time. Cutting out cancer, burning it with radiation, or poisoning it with toxic chemical agents, does not address the underlying problem, but maims, cripples, and destroys the immune system of the cancer victim. If you have cancer, it is very important for you to communicate your ideas, needs, wants, doubts, and questions to your medical team. Those who fare best not only take charge of their health, but actively make choices about their treatment. Consider joining a cancer support group for help; these groups are very beneficial in many ways, and they contribute to increased longevity.

Richard's Story

The story of my patient Richard S. illustrates the importance of a comprehensive approach to health, specifically in the case of prostate cancer.

Richard is 40 years old. He was diagnosed with aggressively metastatic prostate cancer fourteen months ago, which is unusual for such a young man. For approximately three years prior to his diagnosis, Richard's life was wrought with constant and unrelenting stress. Three close family members died, his mother had to be put in a nursing home (he was in charge of selling her house and she lived almost 100 miles away, so there was a lot of driving back and forth), his mother-in-law was diagnosed with Alzheimer's disease, his son was in a serious car wreck, and his wife broke her leg and had to have surgery twice. By the time the third of his close family members and his mother-in-law had died, Richard was already buckling under the pressure. He was seeing a psychologist and a psychiatrist, and was diagnosed with clinical depression.

Then came the really bad news. After experiencing some urinary discomfort, Richard went to his doctor for a physical. The results of the tests couldn't have been worse. His PSA was 22, he was diagnosed with stage D cancer, with a Gleason grading of 8. (Staging of cancer refers to the area and extent of the cancer, A, B, and C representing localized disease, and D denoting the spread of cancer outside the local area to other sites. Grading of cancer is done by looking at the cancer cells under a microscope; well differentiated cells that look most like normal cells are given a grading of 2 to 4, for cells moderately well differentiated, 5 to 7, and poorly differentiated cells are given 8 to 10, and have the worst prognosis.)

With such serious preliminary test results, the next step was for Richard to have a CAT scan to see where the cancer had spread. The CAT scan showed metastasis to the bladder, ureters, and testicles, and also revealed a blood clot in his upper chest area. His doctors convinced him that the blood clot was the greatest threat to his life, so he was hospitalized immediately and put on blood-thinning medication. With time on his hands while undergoing this treatment, Richard began reading books by Bernie Siegel, M.D., Deepak Chopra, M.D., Carl Simington, and others, and these books opened his eyes to many revelations about his life.

Once the blood clot crisis had passed, Richard's doctors recommended twelve months of combined hormone and drug therapy, and eight weeks of radiation treatments, five days a week. After six months of the hormone therapy, Richard refused to continue with it. He not only lost all libido and was unable to have erections, he also experienced memory loss, mood swings, and hot flashes. He says now that he has much more sympathy for menopausal women, because he went through menopause himself! The eight weeks of radiation treatment five days a week caused him to suffer terrible diarrhea and pain.

It was at this point that Richard came to me for help. After comprehensive testing, Richard was found to be mercury toxic, in need of a change in diet, and his colon was infected with some very unfriendly bacteria and parasites. An intensive detoxification program was begun, which included a series of colonic irrigations and significant changes in Richard's diet. He cut way back on fats and sugar, and began taking digestive enzymes and supplements to eliminate the mercury and rebuild his immune system. He also took herbs including Saw palmetto to enhance his healing process, and went for acupuncture treatments to help with the pain that lingered from the radiation.

Richard also began to practice meditation and visualization. For example, he imagined himself being bathed in a golden glowing light and floating in a pool of life-giving water. In this way, he managed to deal with stress and get in touch with his "inner healer".

Richard's other doctors told him it would take six to twelve months to see any effect from the radiation therapy, but after three months of doing the natural therapies just described, and others such as massage and energy work, a repeat scan showed an 85% reduction in all the tumors. The tumor in his bladder was gone and there was no sign of any further metastasis.

Today, five months later, all of Richard's blood tests are normal. His white blood cells are normal, his PSA is normal at 0.3, and all traces of tumors have disappeared. Richard has taken off the twenty extra pounds he had been wanting to lose for the past few years, and he feels great!

Richard believes that the most important aspects of his healing were:

1. He recognized the stress and trauma that had been going on in his life prior to diagnosis, and got help to heal it.

2. He became a major participant in his healing process, making decisions for himself about his treatment, as in the case of refusing another six months of the hormone therapy.

3. He found God, his faith, and his spirituality again.

4. He made radical, but necessary, nutritional changes.

5. He cleansed himself with colonic hydrotherapy and did coffee enemas at home.

6. He sought out acupunture, energy work, and massage.

Of all these steps, Richard feels that next to spirituality, being a participant in his own healing was the most important step in his recovery. Whether facing a fatal disease or just going in for a check-up, you should feel empowered when seeing a physician, not intimidated or frightened into agreeing to a therapy you don't know enough about or don't feel is working. Remember that you always have a choice. Try to make the most informed choices possible so you can stay in charge of your life and your health.

Also remember that a comprehensive, holistic approach to healing—which takes into consideration the whole person, not just an isolated organ, system, or symptom—is the only true path to lasting recovery and wellness.

Conventional Therapies
for Prostate Problems:
What You Need to Know

I T IS IMPORTANT for you to understand that you do have options when undertaking correction of a prostate problem. This book has given you some solid information on the types of therapies employed by naturopathic and holistic healers, and therapies that you can easily incorporate into your daily life. Most medical doctors don't know about them or don't use them, but even in the realm of conventional medicine there are many options for treatment.

The first thing to understand is that if you are having prostate symptoms, it is important to get a diagnosis from a competent physician. Then, get a second and third opinion from a urologist and a holistic practitioner. In this way you can find a treatment that you will feel comfortable with; after all, it is your body.

Although many reports have surfaced showing evidence

of risk factors of a hormonal, familial, environmental, or infectious nature, the only risk factor for prostate cancer agreed upon by medical experts is a high-fat diet. This is now common knowledge, so if your doctor disregards your diet or doesn't ask you anything about it, find another doctor who understands the importance of dietary issues.

Although we know that prostate cancer is becoming more common, cancer historically has proven to be very unpredictable. Seemingly localized disease may spread rapidly, and progressive disease may linger for many years. Why this is so still remains unclear, but some factors may include race, age, and immune system competence. Given the recent statistics for prostate cancer, if a random biopsy were done on 100 men, aged 50 and over, it would show pathological changes that could lead to cancer in 30 to 35 men.

Biopsy is still the most accurate method to detect cancer even though there are risks involved. Biopsies provide the definitive pathological diagnosis and can be fairly easily done. Another test, available since the late 1970s, the PAP for men (Prostatic Acid Phosphatase), is a blood test that is very reliable in identifying an invasive tumor or a metastasis. You may request that more than one pathologist examine and diagnose your sample. Whatever tests or treatments you may choose to undergo, your goal should be to eliminate fear and negativity from your visits to your doctor or surgeon. If you choose surgery, you may request that there be no negative talk during the procedure, that your favorite music be played, and that only positive statements be made regarding your condition, because studies have shown that the recovery rate is better when these parameters have been followed.

• ALLOPATHIC (CONVENTIONAL) TREATMENTS •

Before you can make a decision about treatment for your prostate condition, you must be well-informed. Here are the most common conventional treatments for prostate disease and essential information about each one of them to help you make the best decision possible for your particular situation.

For Prostate Cancer

Prostatectomy—Total surgical removal of the prostate gland, seminal vesicles, and ejaculatory ducts. Some side effects are impotence, incontinence, and dribbling.

Orchiectomy—Removal of the testicles. Although effects are undeniable—no testicles, no testosterone—many men are opposed to such radical therapy.

Cryosurgery—Destruction of the prostate gland by freezing. Studies are inconclusive as to this modality's role in treating prostate cancer.

Radiation—External beam irradiation to the pelvic cavity and prostate or just the prostate after lymphadenectomy (removal of the local lymph nodes). Another technique combines gold seed implants with external beam radiation. Still another option is implantation of radioactive iridium 192 seeds.

There are many negative side effects of radiation: urinary symptoms of frequency, urgency, dysuria (painful urination), hematuria (bloody urine); diarrhea; rectal ulcers, strictures (tightening), fistulas (abscesses with drainage tracts), and proctitis (inflammation of the rectum and anus).

Drug and hormonal therapy—It has been known for 50 years that most prostate cancers are hormone dependent, so the goal of hormone therapy has been to block production or delivery of hormones responsible for the growth of prostate cancer cells. All hormones prescribed are synthetic. Not only are there considerable side-effects and long-term effects associated with their use, but if discontinued, the rebound that follows (re-activation of suppressed hormones) can cause even more problems. The most commonly prescribed drugs and synthetic hormones for prostate cancer are:

- **DES**—Unfortunately, this is the same DES that was mentioned in Chapter 1, and the goal here is basically chemical castration. Side effects are multiple, including nausea, vomiting, edema (swelling), anemia, and cardiovascular complications that can lead to death. Also, external beam localized radiation is performed on the breast tissue to prevent gynecomastia (enlarged breasts), which is painful and unsightly.

- **Progestins**—Given in combination with estrogens (DES) in an attempt to reduce cardiovascular effects. The progestin used in the U.S. is megesterol acetate.

- **Prolactin inhibitors**—The goal here is to stop the production of prolactin by the anterior pituitary gland.

- **L-Dopa** (a drug used to treat Parkinson's disease) is the drug of choice. Side effects include low blood pressure, euphoria, restlessness, and hyperactivity.

- **Anti-androgens**—Flutamide, a nonsteroidal hormonal antagonist, inhibits usage of testosterone in the cells of the prostate. Flutamide blocks the testosterone from binding with its receptor protein, preventing a testosterone effect in the prostate, but serum testosterone is unaffected. Side effects are gynecomastia, nausea, vomiting, abnormal liver function, and elevated serum testosterone (despite the fact that testosterone usage is inhibited, overall testosterone becomes elevated, defeating the purpose of hormonal manipulation). Cyproterone and anadron are also synthetic steroids used in the same way as flutamide. There have been reports of vision disturbances with anadron, so it is under investigational study. Lupron (Leuprolide) is often used in conjunction with flutamide as it inhibits the release of pituitary hormones that stimulate testosterone production in the testes.

- **Androgen synthesis inhibitors** — Ketoconazole, an antifungal drug, blocks the synthesis of testosterone in the testes and adrenal glands in high doses. Side effects are nausea, vomiting, and drug-related liver toxicity. Two other inhibitors of androgen synthesis are spironolactone and aminoglutethimide.

- **Antiestrogens** — Tamoxifen is a nonsteroidal agent that binds estrogen receptors and has been used in female patients with breast cancer. It may block estrogen receptors present in prostate cancer cells. It has been less effective than standard hormonal therapy.

Chemotherapy — This therapy has been disappointing, with remission in only 10 to 15% of cases.

Watchful waiting — This is also a treatment option of doing nothing harmful or invasive, but just monitoring periodically with blood tests and digital rectal exams. Many prostate cancers are slow growing and when doctors find them in older men they usually just do nothing, because the cures can be worse than the disease.

For BPH
Surgical Procedures

TURP— (Transurethral resection of the prostate) A common surgery for BPH in which tiny surgical tools are inserted into the penis and urethra to electrically remove excess prostate tissue. TURP is considered controversial because some authorities believe that this procedure can disseminate (spread) cancer if it is present. This procedure is used with some success in relieving pressure on the prostatic urethra.

TUIP—(Transurethral incision of the prostate) Under local or general anesthesia, one or two incisions are made across the neck of the bladder and prostatic urethra. The incisions are deepened, and the bladder neck and prostatic urethra open, relieving the obstruction. Although complication rates for this surgery are very low, and hospitalization and convalescence greatly diminished compared to the TURP procedure, for some reason it is more rarely used for treating BPH.

Drug Therapy

Proscar (Finasteride)—Until recently, this was the drug of choice for BPH. Unfortunately, it has been shown not only to be ineffective, but that it can actually worsen the symptoms of BPH.

Hytrin (Terazosin)—This long-acting drug, which works by relaxing urinary sphincter spasm, has an additional effect of lowering blood pressure, so for men with hypertension this may be good, but for those with normal blood pressure, dizziness, lightheadedness, or headaches can result. Patients taking Hytrin should be monitored closely.

Other Pharmaceutical Drugs—Drugs similar to those discussed here and other newer drugs are being brought on the market every day. They are too numerous to mention and many are being used in combination with other drugs. Side effects of these drug treatments are basically the same as those described in the previous section.

For Prostatitis

Antibiotic therapy—This is the treatment of choice for most cases of prostatitis. Tetracycline and other antibiotics are used, and some are prescribed for long periods of time at a lower dose.

Natural Testosterone Therapy—A working theory by a European urologist, George Debled, M.D., suggests that testosterone deficiency is more instrumental in the development of BPH and prostatitis than an excess of its by-product, DHT. Dr. Debled was the first doctor to coin the phrase "male andropause," the equivalent in men to a woman's menopause. Although men retain the ability to father children throughout their lives, what andropause represents is a slow but continuous decrease in testosterone, and an increase of the estrogens (remember, men also produce estrogen), sex binding globulin hormones, as well as follicle stimulating hormone, and lutenizing hormone. Dr. Debled takes extensive blood tests on his patients to measure all of these parameters, and prescribes natural testosterone accordingly.

This therapy is worth looking into as an option. Dr. Debled's clinic, which specializes in prostate disorders, has successfully treated thousands of prostate patients. Natural testosterone therapy definitely improves sexual functioning, potency and libido problems, and apparently improves the health of the prostate gland. Dr. Debled claims that he has helped postpone surgical interventions for his patients by ten or more years. Natural testosterone therapy also helps with general drive, not just sex drive, maintaining muscle mass, including the muscles of the prostate gland, promoting a healthier heart and cardiovascular system, and stimulating the immune system.

Natural testosterone may be delivered in various ways— through oral supplementation, a topical cream or patch applied to the scrotum, intramuscular injections, or sublingual pellets. Although a synthetic form of testosterone, called methyl testosterone, has been approved by the FDA, I recommend that you avoid this form. It has been banned in several countries and is linked to liver damage and liver cancer. The natural form is something the body can readily utilize without side-effects.

Whatever treatment you choose, keep in mind that the guidelines for natural treatments given in the previous chapters of this book can help you restore your prostate health.

• REPRODUCTIVE SELF-CARE FOR MEN •

Because prevention and early detection are really the keys to living longer and healthier, women are asked by their physicians to do monthly breast self-exams. By the same token, men can take charge of their health and do two self-exams on a regular basis.

Testicular Self-Exam

The testicular self-exam is simple, painless, and important, particularly for young men between the ages of 15 and 35 because of the increased incidence of testicular cancer in this age group. Although relatively rare, accounting for only 1 percent of all cancers in men, it is one of the most common cancers in men under age 35. If detected early, the cure rate is very high.

The best time to examine your testicles is after a hot bath or shower, when the scrotum is most relaxed. The scrotum regulates the temperature of the testes for optimal sperm production by relaxing away from the body to cool, and drawing up close to the body to heat. The National Cancer Institute recommends that each testicle be examined gently with the fingers of both hands in the following fashion:

1. Place your index and middle fingers on the underside of your testicle and your thumb on top.

2. Then roll your testicle between your thumb and fingers. It should feel firm but not hard, like an earlobe, with some give to it.

3. You should also feel for the epididymis, the storage tube behind each testicle.

With a testicular self-exam, what you want to exclude is the presence of any small, hard, usually painless lump or swelling in either of your testicles. If you feel anything unusual when doing your exam, consult a physician.

Prostate Self-Exam

Although this exam is traditionally done by a physician in a medical office, it is possible for you to do it yourself. A urologist I know told me that some men even do prostate self-massage for chronic prostatitis simply because of the inconvenience and cost of weekly visits to the urologist's office.

It is strongly recommended that men between the ages of 35 and 40 start having yearly digital rectal exams to check prostate health. I realize that prostate self-exams may not be for every man, but for those of you who are willing, and want to know more about your body, the following is for you. To examine your own prostate gland:

1. Insert a lubricated finger—KY jelly works just fine —into the rectum. (You may find that lying on your side with your knees up may be the best position to be in.)

2. You can feel your prostate through the front of your rectum. Be gentle and don't poke at it.

3. You should be able to feel pressure similar to the need to urinate, but this should not be painful. You should be able to scan the entire posterior surface of your prostate with your finger, just like your doctor does when giving you an exam.

4. A healthy prostate should feel like the fleshy part of your hand. It should be about the size of a walnut and have a groove (the median sulcus) down the middle.

5. If you find anything unusual on your self-exam, like hard lumps or increased size, no median sulcus, or even an extremely boggy (or soft) prostate gland, consult a physician.

It is important to remember that the self-exam is not a substitute for a periodic exam by a physician.

———————

I have written this book to help keep you informed about what alternative medicine and conventional medicine have to offer, and about your own body. Being fully informed will make you a healthier person.

ADDITIONAL RESOURCES
FOR NATURAL HEALING

The following information is provided to help you on your healing path. The products, companies, and resources were researched by the author and are of the highest quality, integrity, and purpose.

• PRODUCTS AND MATERIALS •

**PhytoPharmica
aka Enzymatic Therapy**
P.O. Box 1745
Green Bay, WI 54305
1-800-376-7889

Pure, high-quality vitamins, minerals, herbals, and other nutritional supplements and products including high-potency Saw Palmetto and combination prostate formulas. Literature also available.

Uni Key Health Systems, Inc.
P.O. Box 7168
Bozeman, MT 59771
1-800-888-4353

High-quality supplements and creams, as well as literature, from various other companies. This company did its homework to provide the very best available.

Vitality Products
P.O. Box 6237
Olympia, WA 98502
1-800-934-8058

Good nutritional and herbal supplements. Manufacturer of Prostate Nutritional Support, a combination formula containing cranberry extract.

White Lion Trading Company
P.O. Box 11
Chandler, AZ 85224
1-800-755-4324

Herbal remedies. Manufacturers of product called PROST, which is an excellent all-herbal balancing formula.

• LABORATORIES •

*You may have to ask your doctor
to contact these laboratories.*

Analytical Research Laboratories
Endo-Met Laboratories
8650 N. 22nd Ave.
Phoenix, AZ 85021
1-800-848-2667

Tissue analysis with individualized supplement programs with chelated minerals and easily absorbable vitamins.

Doctor's Data Inc.
P.O. Box 111
170 West Roosevelt Road
West Chicago, IL 60185
1-800-323-2784

Particularly good analysis of heavy metals from hair samples and other tissues. Blood, urine, and other tests also analyzed.

TEI (Trace Elements Inc.)
4901 Keller Springs Road
Dallas, TX 75248
1-800-824-2314

Excellent, easy-to-read tissue mineral analysis.

• ORGANIZATIONS, ASSOCIATIONS, •
AND RESOURCES

**American Association of
Naturopathic Physicians
(AANP)**
601 Valley St., Suite 105
Seattle, WA 98109
Referral Line: (206) 298-0125
(206) 298-0126
Fax: (206) 298-0129

**Washington Association of
Naturopathic Physicians
(WANP)**
4224 University Way, Suite J
Seattle, WA 98105
(206) 547-2130
Information Line: 800-438-2882
Fax: (206) 547-2549

American College of Nutrition
722 Robert E. Lee Drive
Wilmington, NC 28412
(910) 452-1222

**Citizens for Alternative
Health Care**
P.O. Box 25312
Seattle, WA 98125-2212
(206) 526-8091
e-mail:
74012.12@compuserve.com

**International Association of
Cancer Victors and Friends**
7740 West Manchester, Suite 110
Playa del Rey, CA 90291
(213) 822-5032

**Cancer Victors and Friends,
Seattle Chapter**
(425) 481-4351
Cancer Victors and Friends,
Apollo Chapter
(educational branch)
President: Albert Schaefer
Al is owner and originator of a
local public access TV program
called Wholesome Voices. He is
also moderator of the Dr. Glenn
Warner Cancer Support Group,
which meets every Wednesday
in Bellevue, WA, and is the direc-
tor of the Health Resources Center of Bellevue, (206) 286-6623.

Herb Research Foundation
1007 Pearl Street, Suite 200
Boulder, CO 80302
(303) 449-2265
Provides research materials on
herbs for consumers, pharma-
cists, physicians, scientists, and
industry.

Mind/Body Health Sciences, Inc.
393 Dixon Road
Boulder, CO 80302
Helps groups organize workshops and provides expert speakers on meditation and mind/body medicine.

Well Being Journal
Editor: Scott Miners
P. O. Box 1542
North Bend, WA 98045-1542
(206) 919-9089 or
(206) 888-9393
Fax: (206) 888-0375
Access all issues of Well Being Journal on the World Wide Web at http://wbj.com

Well Mind Association
4649 Sunnyside N.
Seattle, WA 98105
(206) 547-6167

Dr. Devi S. Nambudripad, D.C., L.Ac.,Ph.D.
N.A.R.F. (Nambudripad's Allergy Research Foundation)
Pain Clinic
6714 Beach Blvd.
Buena Park, CA 90621
714-523-0800
Fax: 714-523-3068

RECOMMENDED READING

• NATURAL HEALING •

Balch, James F., M.D. and Balch, Phyllis A., C.N.C. *Prescription for Nutritional Healing*. New York: Avery Publishing Group, 1990

Bieler, Henry G., M.D. *Food is Your Best Medicine*. New York: Random House, 1965.

Carlson, Richard, Ph.D., and Shield, Benjamin. *Healers on Healing*. Los Angeles: Jeremy P. Tarcher, Inc., 1989.

Cousens, Gabriel, M.D. *Spiritual Nutrition and the Rainbow Diet*. Boulder, CO: Cassandra Press, 1986.

D'Adamo, Peter J., and Catherine Whitney. *Eat Right for Your Type*. New York: G.P. Putnam's Sons, 1996.

Golan, Ralph, M.D. *Optimal Wellness*. New York: Ballantine Books, 1995.

Hay, Louise L. *You Can Heal Your Life*. Carson, CA: Hay House, Inc., 1984.

Murray, Michael, N.D. and Pizzorno, Joseph, N.D. *Encyclopedia of Natural Medicine*. Rocklin, CA: Prima Publishing, 1990.

• MIND/BODY MEDICINE •

Borysenko, Joan, M.D. *Minding the Body, Mending the Mind*. Reading, MA: Addison-Wesley Publishing Company, 1987.

Cousins, Norman. *Anatomy of an Illness*. New York: W.W. Norton, 1979.

Dossey, Larry, M.D. *Space, Time and Medicine*. Boston: Shambala Publications, 1982.

• MIND POWER •

Howard, Vernon. *Psychopictography*. West Nyack, NY: Parker Publishing Co., Inc., 1965.

____. *The Mystic Path To Cosmic Power*. West Nyack, NY: Parker Publishing Co., Inc., 1967.

• REFLEXOLOGY •

Bergson, Anika and Tuchack, Vladimir. *Zone Therapy*. Denver: The Nutri-Books Corp., 1974.

Carter, Mildred. *Helping Yourself with Foot Reflexology*. West Nyack, NY: Parker Publishing Co., Inc., 1969.

____. *Body Reflexology*. West Nyack, NY: Parker Publishing Co., Inc., 1983.

Marquardt, Hanne. *Reflex Zone Therapy of the Feet*. Wellingborough Northamptonshire, England: Thorsons Publishers Limited, 1983.

• HERBAL MEDICINE •

Hoffman, David. *The Herb User's Guide*. Wellingborough Northamptonshire, England: Thorsons Publishing Group, 1987.

____. *The Holistic Herbal*. Longmead Shaftsbury Dorset, England: Element Books Limited, 1988.

REFERENCES

Albin, Steve, N.D., Gary Burr, N.D, and Prudence Broadwell, N.D. *Notes on Natural Therapeutics from Lectures of Dr. John Bastyr.* Bastyr College, 1977.

American Cancer Society. *Cancer Facts and Figures,* 1994.

American Society of Nutritional Research. *The Prostate Gland.* Research Bulletin 190.

Brown, Donald N.D. Men's Health Survey Shows Men Worried and Confused About Prostate Problems—Latest Breakthroughs Are Unknown To Most! *Journal of Longevity Research* 3:1, 1997.

Center for Science in the Public Interest. T*he Cancer Men Don't Talk About.* Nutrition Action Newsletter 20:2, March 1993.

Center for Science in the Public Interest. *For Men Only.* Nutrition Action Newsletter 22:5, June 1995.

Guyton, Dr. Arthur C. *Textbook of Medical Physiology,* Seventh Edition. Philadelphia: W.B. Saunders Co., 1986.

Hoag, J. M., D.O. "Disorders of the Male Genitourinary System." In *Osteopathic Medicine,* 666-75. New York: McGraw-Hill Book Company, 1969.

Better Prostate Cancer Predictions. *Johns Hopkins Medical Letter* 6:7, September 1994.

Kellogg, J. H., M.D., LL.D., F.A.C.S. *Rational Hydrotherapy—A manual of the physiological and therapeutic effects of hydriatic procedures, and the technique of their application in the treatment of disease.* Modern Medicine Publishing Company, 1923.

Krezeski, T., M. Kazon, A. Borkowski, A. Witeska and J. Kuczera. Combined extracts of urtica dioica and pygeum africanum in the treatment of benign prostatic hyperplasia: double blind comparison of two doses. *Clinical Therapeutics* 15-6:1012, 1993.

Lepor, H, and Rigaud, G. The Efficacy of Transurethral Resection of the Prostate in Men with Moderate Symptoms of Prostatism. *Journal of Urology* 143:533-537, 1990.

Lobay, Douglas, N.D. For Men Only—Getting Serious About Some Very Important Aspects of Your Health. *Country Health* 13:4, July/August 1995.

Mann, C. C. The Prostate Cancer Dilemma. *The Atlantic Monthly* 102-118, November 1993.

Oesterling, J. E. Benign Prostatic Hyperplasia: Medical and Minimally Invasive Treatment Options. *New England Journal of Medicine* 332:2, 99-109, January 12, 1995.

Pizzorno, Joseph, N.D. and Murray, Michael, N.D. "Serenoa Reopens." In *A Textbook of Natural Medicine*. Seattle: JBC Publications, 1989.

PSA Test: How Well Does It Detect Prostate Cancer? *University of California at Berkeley Wellness Letter* 9:11, August 1993.

Richards-Griffen, Hazel S. *92 Years Perfect Health in an Unpolluted Body*. Revised edition of *Science of Perfect Health*. Orlando, Florida: Words-To-Go, 1995.

Rittmaster, R. S. Finasteride. *New England Journal of Medicine* 330:120-125, 1994.

Swanson, Mark, N.D. The Treatment of Benign Prostatic Hyperplasia (BPH): Phyto-Synergist Extracts of Saw Palmetto, Pygeum Africanum, and Unrefined Pumpkin Oil. In *The Good Doctor—For Doctors*.

Williams, Stephen. Managing Your Prostate: A Man's Guide. *Prevention*. April 1986.

Windsor, Dr. James C. The Body/Mind/Spirit Connection. *United States Psychotronics Association Newsletter* 14:2, Spring 1996.

Woolf, Steven H., M.D.,M.P.H. Current Concepts: Screening for Prostate Cancer with Prostate Specific Antigen. *New England Journal of Medicine* 333:21, November 23, 1995.

Zubay, Geoffrey. "Complex Lipids, The Eicosanoids: Prostaglandins, Thromboxanes, Leukotrienes, and Hydroxy-Eicosaenoic Acids." In *Biochemistry*, Second Edition. New York: MacMillan Publishing Co., 1988.

INDEX

5-alpha reductase, 6

A vitamin, 33, 35
AANP. *See* Naturopathic Physicians, American Association of (AANP)
abscesses with drainage tracts, 81
ACES, 33
acids, fatty, 34-35
acupuncture, 77-78
acute cystitis, treatments for, 51-52
acute prostatitis, 3-4
addiction to drugs, treatments for, 50
adrenal glands, 15
affirmations for healing, 67-69
African Americans, risk of getting prostate cancer, 8
African evergreen tree, 39
aging, as cause of rising PSA levels, 2
alanine, 34, 35
alcohol
consumption of, 10
treatments for alcoholism, 50
allergies
allergy elimination technique, 14-15
food allergy test, 14-15
from food, 12
allopathic treatments for prostate problems, 79-86
alternate baths, 47-48, 51-52
alternate salad dressing recipe, 20
alternating sitz baths, 47-48, 51-52
aluminum, 74
American diet, 9
American ginseng, 41
amino acid chelate, 30
amino acids, 34
aminoglutethimide, 83
anadron, 83
analyses
of blood, 14
of hair, 14-15, 30, 73-74
Analytical Research Laboratories, 90
Anatomy of an Illness, 64
anatomy of prostate, 1
androgen synthesis inhibitors, 83
andropause in males, 85
anemia, 82

anger, effects on prostate health, 64
angina, 41
animal protein, 13
anterior pituitary gland, 82
anti-androgens, 82-83
antibiotic therapies, 85
antiestrogens, 83
antifungal drugs, 83
antioxidants
reduced L-Glutathione, 74
selenium, 31, 33
vitamin A, 33, 35
vitamin C, 33-34, 35
antiseptics for urinary tract, 38, 42
anus, inflammation of rectum and, 81
anxiety, effects on prostate health, 64
aphrodisiac, 40
Arctostaphylos uva ursi, 39
arsenic, 74
arteriosclerosis and hot foot baths, 53
Asians, risk of getting prostate cancer, 8
associations for natural healing, 91-92
astringents, 39, 42
attitudes, effects on prostate health, 64

B-6 vitamin, 32-33, 35
B-complex vitamins, 33, 35
bacteria, as cause of prostatitis, 4
balancers of hormones, 38
baths, 46-56
beans, 15
bearberry, 39
bedwetting, treatments for, 51
bee pollen, 43
beer consumption, 6, 10
benign prostatic hyperplasia. See BPH
berries, juniper, 42
beta-carotene, 33
biopsies, 7, 80
bladder
bladder points (reflex), 49, 62
bladder sphincter, 43
treatments for bladder problems, 42, 52, 84
blitz guss, 50-52
blood
and calcium supplements, 32

97